CW01333185

Turn Yourself On

Turn Yourself On

Anna Hushlak, DPhil,
with Billie Quinlan

Founders of Ferly

PENGUIN LIFE

AN IMPRINT OF

PENGUIN BOOKS

PENGUIN LIFE

UK | USA | Canada | Ireland | Australia
India | New Zealand | South Africa

Penguin Life is part of the Penguin Random House group of companies whose addresses can be found at global.penguinrandomhouse.com

Penguin Random House UK,
One Embassy Gardens, 8 Viaduct Gardens, London SW11 7BW

penguin.co.uk

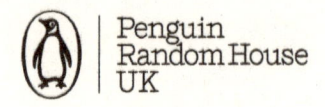

Penguin Random House UK

First published 2025

001

Copyright © Anna Hushlak and Billie Quinlan, 2025

The moral right of the authors has been asserted

Material from *Burnout* by Emily Nagoski and Amelia Nagoski published by Vermilion. Copyright © Emily Nagoski and Amelia Nagoski, 2020. Reprinted by permission of the Random House Group Limited.

Material from *Come Together* by Emily Nagoski published by Vermilion. Copyright © Emily Nagoski, 2024. Reprinted by permission of the Random House Group Limited.

The authors and publisher gratefully acknowledge the permission granted to reproduce the copyright material in this book. Every effort has been made to trace copyright holders and to obtain their permission. The publisher apologizes for any errors or omissions and, if notified of any corrections, will make suitable acknowledgement in future reprints or editions of this book.

No part of this book may be used or reproduced in any manner for the purpose of training artificial intelligence technologies or systems. In accordance with Article 4(3) of the DSM Directive 2019/790, Penguin Random House expressly reserves this work from the text and data mining exception.

Set in 13.3/15.8pt Garamond MT Pro
Typeset by Jouve (UK), Milton Keynes
Printed and bound in Great Britain by Clays Ltd, Elcograf S.p.A.

The authorized representative in the EEA is Penguin Random House Ireland, Morrison Chambers, 32 Nassau Street, Dublin D02 YH68

A CIP catalogue record for this book is available from the British Library

ISBN: 978–0–241–70664–0

Penguin Random House is committed to a sustainable future for our business, our readers and our planet. This book is made from Forest Stewardship Council® certified paper.

MIX
Paper | Supporting responsible forestry
FSC® C018179

For every woman who has been made to feel small,
has worried about being normal,
or has ever felt shame
– this is for you.

This is your invitation –
to (re)discover your sense of aliveness,
to connect to yourself and the world around you,
and to cultivate the fullest and most powerful version of you.

Contents

A Note from Billie   ix
Introduction   1

Principle 1 – Assert Your Agency   17
Principle 2 – Balance Your Power   51
Principle 3 – Build Your Self-Confidence   91
Principle 4 – Cultivate Your Intimacy   123
Principle 5 – Embrace Your Desire   158
Principle 6 – Honour Your Health   192
Principle 7 – Prioritize Your Pleasure   232
Principle 8 – Improve Your Communication   270

Conclusion   313
Will you help us empower more women?   323
Acknowledgements   325
Notes   327
Index   349

A Note from Billie

In October 2015, aged twenty-four, I was sexually assaulted at work (more on this later in the book).

For the next eighteen months, shame, self-loathing and a fear of my own sexuality would haunt me. Back then, I didn't even know that what had happened was considered assault, and so I struggled to understand why it was having such a big impact on me. I felt pathetic, and like a silly little girl who couldn't handle a bit of office banter.

A year after the assault, every part of my life was suffering. It was during one of these relentless days that an email hit my inbox, with the subject line 'Escape the City'. I opened it and discovered a three-month programme that would help guide me through a career transition. I signed up right away and got so much more out of it than I could have hoped for. I not only discovered my passion for health and working with women, I also developed a newfound sense of confidence and community. After completing the programme, I quit my job and studied to become a health coach, through which I started working with female clients to help them improve their wellbeing and overall quality of life. During this time, a friend sent me a job posting. A start-up incubator (Zinc VC) was recruiting people passionate about transforming the lives of women and girls globally.

Deep within my body, I felt this overwhelming pull to apply.

Suddenly, everything I had been through took on a new and profound purpose, as if it had prepared me for the journey I was about to embark on and the women I was going to help. I joined Zinc VC in October 2017, two years after my assault.

I was so excited to start the incubator and spent the first two weeks of the programme alongside forty-nine other mission-driven people in the council's office in King's Cross, London. The venue was old and unloved but quite spectacular in its own way. It had a grand staircase and a magnificent atrium. Day after day, we sat under that glass ceiling while a broad array of experts gave us detailed presentations to prepare us for our work supporting women around the world. We learned about everything from menopause to schizophrenia and urban planning to financial health. Seemingly, all areas of women's mental and emotional wellbeing were covered. Well, except one critical pillar: sexual wellbeing. With every passing expert, I thought to myself, surely today we'll have a guest speak to us about women's sexuality. But no such luck.

On the final day of the presentations, we introduced ourselves to the rest of the cohort and shared any reflections we'd had so far. I was so nervous about speaking. I felt like such an imposter in this room of accomplished people. I was so distracted thinking about what I was going to say, I barely listened to anyone's introduction until I heard this confident, excitable, warm, Canadian voice booming out over the room. I looked up and it was love at first sight. This woman, with her blonde hair and warm smile, had me hooked on every word. 'Hi,' she said, 'I'm Anna Hushlak...'

Instantly, I knew I wanted to be her friend, but more importantly, I wanted to change the world with her. After our introductions, we broke for lunch. A bunch of us sat down together and started discussing the last two weeks. I mentioned how strange it was that no one had come to talk to us about the sexual challenges women were facing and the impact this was having on their mental and emotional health. A few people nodded and then I turned to Anna. We locked eyes, banged our fists on the table and exploded into a heated discussion on how absurd it was. I shared my assault with Anna and she shared her own experience of surviving sexual violence. This is where Ferly's story begins, with a pair of fired-up, angry women united by a shared purpose.

Building a business with someone you've only just met is a little bonkers. Like getting married after your first date. For our partnership to succeed, it required significant nurturing, intimacy and trust. So, over the next few months, while we built Ferly through thousands of customer interviews, product brainstorms, branding workshops and expert reviews, we also built our co-founder relationship in less orthodox ways. Competitive white-water rafting, naked showers together, pumpkin carving, sleepovers and erotica readings. We came *very* close to getting matching clitoris tattoos on our index fingers, but the shop wasn't open. There's still time though ;)

But while our relationship flourished, Ferly was hitting hurdle after hurdle.

As we started building the business, the taboo nature of female sexuality reared its ugly head. Various mentors pushed back. They told us that female sexual difficulties (e.g. anorgasmia, low libido, vulvodynia, vaginismus, etc.) – issues that affect 51 per cent of women – weren't a real or meaningful enough problem for us to solve.*

We were also told we needed a more 'diverse' team. When we asked what they meant by 'diverse', the answer was: 'A male co-founder.' Most of our advisors discouraged us from pursuing the business as two female founders, especially two who were trying to solve a 'niche' problem. They told us we'd have a hard time securing funding.

We ignored their advice and soldiered on.

On the last day of the programme, we pitched to external investors. Before going on stage, an older man in our cohort said the only reason we'd get funding was because I was seducing them by wearing heels and red lipstick. He called us the 'Blow Job Girls'. After the pitch, another cohort member said my voice was 'too sexy' and suggested I adjust it, so as not to make men in the audience uncomfortable.

---

* Anorgasmia is when a person regularly struggles to orgasm despite sexual stimulation. It's much more common for women and is often mental and emotional, not necessarily physical. Vulvodynia is persistent pain in the vulva that does not have an identifiable cause and has lasted three or more months. Vaginismus is pain with penetration and the sudden tightening of muscles in the vagina, and is often psychosomatic. For more info, check out the Vaginismus Network.

A NOTE FROM BILLIE

As it turned out, we were the first team on the programme to secure a term sheet (investment). Lucky for us, it also happened to be from an amazing female investor.

However, she then had to battle the firm's vice clause. This prevented investments in sex, gambling and drugs. Ferly, a digital therapy app for female sexual wellbeing, was being lumped into the same category as hardcore porn and class A drugs.

After months of hard work, we launched Ferly. We were quickly approached by Apple, who wanted to feature us as 'App of the Day'. It was so exciting to receive the recognition and felt like progress at long last. Our excitement was short-lived. Less than twenty-four hours later, Apple kicked us off the App Store (and Google booted us off the Play Store too). Apparently, our abstract collage imagery and use of the words 'desire' and 'arousal' were too explicit. For what would be the first of many times, we were banned due to 'company policy'.

Since going live with the Ferly app in 2019, together Anna and I have been at war. Fighting against investors, big tech, censorship and media bans, misogyny and sexism. We faced so many challenges launching Ferly. Can you guess the biggest one of all?

Shame.

There is so much shame around human sexuality, especially female sexuality. This stops us from talking honestly about our wants, needs and experiences. We're afraid we'll be judged if we speak openly, and question whether anyone will still love us if we share the deepest and most intimate parts of ourselves. But, as the great Dr Brené Brown teaches us in her famous TED talk, the antidote to shame is vulnerability.[1]

Throughout the process of building Ferly, Anna and I have been so inspired by the women who've had the courage to share their stories – and to do so with their whole hearts. Even more inspiring is witnessing their transformation once they do. To honour these women, and to encourage more of you to do the same, Anna and I are about to share our own stories with you. The stories in this book are us at our most vulnerable and most exposed. It's scary to put them out there, but we're not ashamed of the women we are – just as you shouldn't be either. Coming back to Brené, she argues that allowing ourselves to be vulnerable is the birthplace of not only joy but also creativity, belonging and love. This has certainly been our experience.

The last seven years have been an immense period of personal growth. When we set out to build a sexual wellbeing company, Anna and I had no idea about the journey we would find ourselves on. Owning our sexuality, ridding ourselves of shame and fully accepting the women we are has unlocked opportunities and experiences we could only ever dream of. We learned how to share, find our aliveness again, and turn ourselves on, so we can flourish in the bedroom and beyond.

Are you ready?

Because now, it's your turn.

I want to publicly and loudly acknowledge my incredible friend, Dr Anna Hushlak. She is a phenomenal researcher and has somehow managed to take all our learnings, combine them with the science on sex and women's health, and write this book in a way that is practical, empowering and a joy to read. The love I have developed for this woman over the last seven years is deep and profound. So, my ultimate learning is this: if you want a truly rewarding love affair, find women you can shower with (like we did in the first week we met) while discussing all the ways you get pleasure from sex and from life, and hold those friendships tight. When women come together and share openly, magic happens.

'Who are *you*?' said the Caterpillar.

This was not an encouraging opening for a conversation. Alice replied, rather shyly, 'I – I hardly know, sir, just at present – at least I know who I *was* when I got up this morning, but I think I must have been changed several times since then.'

— Lewis Carroll, *Alice's Adventures in Wonderland*

Introduction

This is a book for any woman who wants to have a better sex life.

It's also about a lot more than that though; this is a book about self-discovery – *your* self-discovery. It's about diving into the amazing world of you. Because believe it or not, sex is never, ever just physical. It's not something you do, it's something you feel, and how you feel about it matters. We'd argue it matters more than the act itself. By the end of this book, you'll not only have the tools you need to cultivate a great sex life; you'll also know how to cultivate the most important relationship you'll ever have – the one you have with yourself.

Your sexuality is a powerful force in how you show up for yourself and in the world. Embracing it means unlocking the most authentic version of you. Accessing your authenticity might come from tuning into your senses and being mindful of how eroticism appears in your everyday life. It might come from feeling confident asserting your boundaries and advocating for your needs. It might be anything! Whether you like it or not, you can't – and shouldn't – leave your sexual self at the bedroom door. When you're empowered sexually, a deep-rooted sense of self-worth and confidence spills over into every other aspect of your life.

First things first, before we get into any of that, close your eyes and picture your sex life. Think about some of the stuff that might come with it. This could be intimacy, desire, pleasure, novelty, confidence, communication . . .

Now, think about where you're currently at and how you might make your sex life better. How confident are you, on a scale from 1 to 10, in the steps you need to take to improve it? (With 1 being 'No idea' and 10 being 'Totally got this'.)

Picked your number? Great!

Jot it down somewhere for you to come back to later – on this page, on your phone or send yourself an email. And remember, there's no right or wrong answer here. This is just a reference point for you to return to as you set out on your journey to better sex.

If you're picking up this book, it's probably because you're ready to explore your sexual self, kick things up a notch in the bedroom or feel more sexually empowered. Whatever the reason(s), welcome! Whether you're in the 51 per cent of women who are currently struggling with sex and feel a bit stuck, or you're happy with your sex life and are looking for a little extra zing, we're super pleased you're here.

When it comes to empowering you to have healthy, confident and pleasurable sex, Billie and I have got it covered. That's why we often get messages like these from women we've worked with, whose transformations have been magical:

- *'I feel so in tune with my body now. I wish all women everywhere could experience these breakthroughs.'*

INTRODUCTION

- *'Yesterday, after years of limiting beliefs around masturbation, I had my first orgasm (& then my second)! You are my heroes!!! NEVER STOP DOING WHAT YOU'RE DOING!'*
- *'I've been struggling with trauma-induced sex aversion, but thanks to you, me and my partner managed intimacy for the first time in 5 years last night! Thank you!!'*
- *'You've shown me how much the mind influences desire and pleasure and how to identify my inner sexual critic. I feel so much more confident and closer to my true self.'*
- *'I now understand how my thoughts affect my libido and what I need to feel in the mood. This work is amazing, I'm so grateful for it!'*

See? Your sex life might feel complicated, but it doesn't have to. Over the years, we've had the chance to help many, many women – seriously, over half a million! – improve their sex lives. Chances are, if you're here, you probably have some of the same goals they did:

- Better relationships and deeper intimacy
- More confidence in bed
- Knowing and understanding your desires
- Being present and connected during sex
- Expressing your sexual needs
- Enjoying pleasure and orgasms too
- Feeling comfortable talking about sex

Does any of this hit home? If so, you're exactly where you need to be.

Here's an exercise to get you started: answer the three questions below. The key is to be honest with yourself. These questions will help you define what you want to get from this book, and where you're at right now. We'd recommend using a notebook or the notes app on your phone for this (and for the many other exercises within this book).

1. My definition of 'good sex' is . . .
2. Over the course of this book, I'd like to learn . . .
3. When I think about unpacking my sex life, the words that most describe how I'm feeling are . . .

Now, about that last question in the exercise – sex can stir up a whole mix of emotions. It's okay to feel a bit anxious, sceptical, shy or even embarrassed. But by picking up this book, we hope you're also feeling curious, hopeful and excited by what might be possible.

We get it, because we've been there too, and it's why we can't wait to be on this journey with you.

Who we are and why we wrote this book

Hey there! If we haven't met yet, I'm Anna, the author and narrator of this book. Of course, I could not

INTRODUCTION

have done this work without significant contributions, insights and ideas from my fabulous co-author, co-founder and best friend, Billie. Consider us your new ride-or-dies in your journey to better sex. We'll say it straight up, we're not therapists or medical doctors (but I do have a doctorate and know a thing or two about research). What we've got is a solid track record in navigating the world of all-things-sex. Our expertise comes in large part from our own real-life rocky rides. From a lack of Sex Ed in school, to surviving sexual violence and sexual assault in the workplace, to ultimately helping more than 500,000 women worldwide have a more satisfying time between the sheets.

We're the brains behind Ferly, one of the first digital sexual wellbeing companies for women. We started Ferly because we were done with the shame and stigma clouding women's pleasure. We'd battled from the trenches of underwhelming sex ourselves and we wanted something better, not just for us but for everyone.

When it comes to sex, there's a lot of concern about being 'normal'. If you've ever felt like you're struggling in the bedroom, you might have worried something's 'off' or you're not quite 'normal'. This can lead to feeling like you're broken or you need fixing. But here's the thing – we're giving 'normal' a bit of a makeover. In this book, when we talk about 'normal', we're talking about what's common, typical or usual. And for us, it's about asking, 'What even is "normal", anyway?'

Here's an example: society's got this annoying idea that it's 'normal' for women to settle for less-than-great sex.

Spoiler alert: it's not.

Supposedly, women are 30 per cent less likely to orgasm than men during heterosexual sex[1] – that's considered 'normal'. And yet, during solo play, they orgasm 92–95 per cent of the time, so is it?

And yeah, one in two women is likely to experience low desire at some point in their lives – that's 'normal'. But then again, we've been fed a bunch of lies about all desire being spontaneous, so is it?

Here's a little secret: pretty much everything Billie and I thought we knew about sex was wrong. And we're guessing a lot of what you've heard might be wrong too.

When we started Ferly, we were new to the whole 'sex' thing. Sure, we'd been having it, we knew the basics, but the nitty-gritty details? Not so much. We didn't know the difference between a vagina and a vulva, let alone what a clitoris looked like (no worries if you're in the same boat – that's exactly why you're here!).

We were over the shame and taboos surrounding sex, pleasure and our bodies. We were tired. Tired of overthinking, struggling with orgasms, dealing with low desire, failing to express ourselves sexually and feeling unsexy.

When we look back to why we struggled with enjoying sex, it's finally clear.

Sex is about so much more than sex. It's a reflection of who you are and how you value yourself. Your sexual wellbeing is as much a part of your health as your physical, emotional or mental wellbeing. Yet many of us don't see it this way. That's because (for no good reason) it's still so taboo, leaving many of us feeling ashamed both in and out of the bedroom.

INTRODUCTION

Dr Brené Brown describes shame as the gut-wrenching feeling and belief that we're not enough and we're unworthy of love and connection.[2] Shame is more than feeling guilty or messing up; it's believing something is fundamentally wrong with you.[3]

Shame is real.

In fact, it's so real that in a review of eighteen studies looking at how shame shows up in the brain, neuroscientists found it activates our pain network, meaning we can even experience it as physical pain.[4] It's no wonder it has an impact on how we think and feel about sex.

Over the years, we've heard countless stories about the shadow shame casts across people's lives. We've felt its weight ourselves too. It hovers and follows you around, making you doubt everything from your desires to your bodies to your experiences – or lack thereof. The sad truth is we're ashamed of all sorts of things, especially when it comes to sex.

But here's the deal: Billie and I are done with it, and you can be too.

Billie, as a certified health coach, and me, as an academic researcher and social scientist, decided it was time to kick shame to the curb, and break free from taboos around sex and pleasure. We also wanted to finally understand how to have great sex. Since launching Ferly in 2019, we have hit both of those objectives and we've learned far more than we'd bargained for.

From speaking to hundreds of experts about the psychology, physiology and neurobiology of sex, to practising tantra and somatic bodywork, to exploring how to take back control in the bedroom, we've learned having great sex is far from where it ends. Our own journeys, alongside the transformations of thousands of others, have shown us that sex isn't just something you do but a gateway to your own self-discovery. By understanding what you believe, what you like (and what you don't) and what brings you meaning, as well as how to ask for what you want, you start to learn who you really are, not just beneath the sheets but in the rest of your life too.

This book is a culmination of everything we've learned so far, all wrapped up in eight principles. These principles are key to helping you have healthy, confident and pleasurable sex – and to lead a more joyful and fulfilling life overall. That's why we're here, and why we wrote this book. We're sharing these eight principles for two reasons. First, because we want to provide women with the support we wish we'd had, but never got. Second, because we truly believe they will help you have a better sex life and discover what turns you on, so you can find your power both in and out of the bedroom.

What is sexual wellbeing, and why should you care?

Alright, let's look at what good sex and sexual health *actually* means, shall we? The World Health Organization (WHO), has a great definition:

INTRODUCTION

> A state of physical, emotional, mental and social wellbeing in relation to sexuality; it is not merely the absence of disease, dysfunction or infirmity. Sexual health requires a positive and respectful approach to sexuality and sexual relationships, as well as the possibility of having pleasurable and safe sexual experiences, free of coercion, discrimination and violence. For sexual health to be attained and maintained, the sexual rights of all persons must be respected, protected and fulfilled.[5]

Now, there are three biggies we need to unpack here, because they each have a huge influence on your sex life – and, honestly, your life as a whole.

First, having positive sexual health and wellbeing is your right. Think about it: some things are so essential they're considered basic rights, like education or rest. Health, wellbeing and pleasure are right up there too – alongside liberty, social justice and equality. These aren't the cherries on top; they're the whole sundae.

Second, wellbeing isn't just about your body – it also encompasses your mind, relationships and culture. It's like looking at a painting – you need to step back to see the whole picture, not just focus on one corner. This is where the biopsychosocial-cultural model comes in. This fancy term basically means we need to look at everything from our biology (like hormones and genetics), to our psychology (like our thoughts and feelings about sex), our social interactions (like how we communicate with our partners) and our cultural background (like the beliefs and values we've grown up with).

Here's a real-life example for you: Imagine your sexual desire has dipped and seems to be taking a little vacation. Biologically, it could be due to hormone imbalances. Psychologically, stress and anxiety might be crashing the party. Socially, maybe a recent argument with your partner is putting a dampener on things. And culturally, those pesky societal taboos around what desire is 'supposed' to look like could be throwing a spanner in the works. It could be one of these, a mix, or even all of them! That's why we use the biopsychosocial-cultural model – to look at everything going on rather than just zeroing in on the stuff to do with your body.

Third, good sex is way more than the absence of problems. Saying sex is good because there are no problems is like saying a meal is good because it didn't make you sick. Let's be honest here, folks, we're aiming higher than 'avoiding food poisoning'. Good sex is sex that feels good *and more*. Think of your sexual wellbeing like your physical wellbeing. Being well doesn't just mean not being sick. It means feeling good in your body, being full of energy and doing what you love. It's also about not waiting until something goes wrong to fix it. A lot of us only pay attention to our wellbeing or our health when we're ill rather than learning how to avoid getting ill in the first place. Billie and I want to challenge this way of thinking, and help you be proactive, so you can transform your life from good to great, in and out of the bedroom.

INTRODUCTION

What this book is, what it's not and how it's organized

Think of this book as your go-to toolkit, not just a bedtime story. Sure, you're meant to read it, but you're also meant to put it to work. It's designed for action – not for flipping through. It's a guide for improving not only your sex life, but your life in general. Sex is pretty personal, right? So, this book should be too. Here's a little nudge: make this book your own. Highlight passages that hit home, scribble notes in the margins, dog-ear pages. Do whatever helps you return to the bits you need when you need them. Consider this book a road map that keeps you coming back – equipped and ready for whatever comes your way.

This book isn't about quick fixes, it's about real tools for real life. It's here to guide you through understanding your *relationship* with sex, not the mechanics of how to do it. Each chapter is a step forward, helping you discover what turns you on, both in sex and in life. We've filled these pages with real stories, science and practical tools to put these principles into play. Each chapter follows the same structure, making it easy to follow and even easier to revisit whenever you need a refresher. Within them, we'll cover one of the eight principles, a case study from our own lives, a dose of science, and three practical tools to help you apply that principle in real life. We've also included downloadable tools, extra resources and templates for you at www.turnyourselfon.co.

Now, you might have picked up this book looking for quick tips or hoping to find the answers to big questions, like 'how to be more confident in bed', 'how to increase desire' or 'how to have an orgasm'. Hang tight – we're diving into all that. But remember, great sex starts with you – mentally and emotionally, not just physically. To get the most out of your sex life, you need to first understand your personal relationship with sex. This means making sense of what it looks like, where it comes from and how it's impacting you, for better or worse. Think of it like building a house: if your foundation isn't solid, the whole thing risks falling apart.

So, while you might be tempted to skip ahead to the chapters that catch your eye, try to resist. Reading this book from start to finish will build that strong foundation for you, brick by brick. But if you're eager to jump to a specific chapter, go for it – just make sure to circle back and cover all the essentials.

And a heads-up: the first two chapters include some graphic content. We debated whether to include these stories as they are a little heavier, but we decided they were too important to omit. They're part of our truths, and they also represent real-life experiences that many of us have had to navigate in one form or another. Sharing them is a step towards shedding our own feelings of shame and challenging the taboos and silence head-on. We'll let you know when those parts are coming up, so feel free to skip them if you want.

INTRODUCTION

Some things you might want to know

When we chose the stories for this book, we wanted to share them in a way that was unfiltered, vulnerable and honest. All of them are real. In writing Billie's experiences, I've aimed to capture them exactly as she explained them to me. Yet, like with any memory, they get fuzzier with time and may be imperfect. What we have shared is to the best of our knowledge – it's how we remember it. We've also changed everyone's names and identifying details for privacy. Putting ourselves out there has taken courage and a little bit of reassurance too. It goes to show we all need it sometimes. Both Billie and I felt uneasy – guilty even – for taking up space and using language we didn't feel was ours to claim.

But here's the thing: shame loves to hide in the shadows.

Together, when we bring all of our stories into the light, we take a collective stand against shame. It's all about connecting, with ourselves and each other, and realizing none of us is alone. By opening up, our hope is to help you navigate your own experiences, like others have done for us by sharing theirs.

Next up, we've packed this book with science, but don't worry, it's anything but a textbook. We're talking psychology, sex science, neurobiology and more, all researched and written by some great leaders in the field. In identifying the eight principles, we've handpicked the research insights that were game changers for us (and the thousands of women we've worked with). We've also shared some of the science that forms the foundation of each one. That being said, we couldn't fit it all in. So, if you're a fellow science nerd like me, check out the resources at the end of each chapter for a deeper dive.

It's also important to flag that while science is amazing, it doesn't always get everything right. This is especially true when it comes to women's health and pleasure, where it's gotten a lot wrong. For example, research has been pretty focused on cisgender women. But, thanks to more diverse voices in science shaking up our understanding of sex and sexuality, change is in the air.

And hey, although Billie and I have written this book for women, it's not only women who should read it. Understanding and making sense of each other's bodies and experiences makes the world a richer place. Think of it as an opportunity to help close the pleasure gap. We write from our own perspectives as women, so the vibe might resonate more with those who identify as female. We're talking about all women here, regardless of the sex you were assigned at birth. But as a heads-up, we're not diving into the specific experiences of trans and non-binary folks. Not because it's not important, but because there are experts from those communities who can speak to those experiences far better than we can.*

---

* Some reads to check out: Dr Julia Serano's *Whipping Girl: A Transsexual Woman on Sexism and the Scapegoating of Femininity*; Dr Laura Erickson-Schroth's *Trans Bodies, Trans Selves: A Resource for the Transgender Community*; Janet Mock's *Redefining Realness: My Path to Womanhood, Identity, Love & So Much More*; Dr Kit Heyam's *Before We Were Trans: A New History of Gender*; Vivek Shraya's *I'm Afraid of Men*; Laura Kate

INTRODUCTION

With that in mind, we also wanted to acknowledge where we're coming from. Both Billie and I are white, cisgender, able-bodied, straight women from middle-class backgrounds with university degrees. Through our stories, you'll hear about our own challenges, but we recognize we've had many advantages and opportunities available to us that aren't there for everyone. Our aim? To make the insights and tools in this book as accessible as possible, so everyone, from any background, can get something out of it.

How this book will benefit you

Growing up, *Alice's Adventures in Wonderland* was one of my favourite reads. Sure, there's much debate on whether it's feminist or anti-feminist, but put that aside for a minute. For me, I saw Alice as an adventurous and assertive character, whose curiosity drove her own journey of self-discovery. I also loved that Wonderland was all in Alice's mind. A world built entirely from the power of her own imagination.

Think of yourself as a sort-of-Alice, and this book as your personal guide down the rabbit hole to discover your sexual self. Your sexuality is a part of who you are, and sex offers a unique peek into your identity. If you've never looked through this window or if you're new to

---

Dale's *Gender Euphoria: Stories of Joy from Trans, Non-Binary and Intersex Writers*; Dr Meg-John Barker and Dr Alex Iantaffi's *Life Isn't Binary: On Being Both, Beyond, and In-Between.*

meeting this part of yourself, you're in for some eye-opening discoveries. The best part? The skills that make for a great sex life – for example, confidence, pleasure and communication – are the same ones that make for a great life overall. It's like using the same ingredients but in new and exciting ways to create different dishes. Master these principles in the bedroom, and tackling challenges like having a difficult conversation or negotiating that well-deserved pay rise will seem like a walk in the park.

As we go through the chapters, we'll guide you through step-by-step instructions on how to enhance your sex life, enrich your overall life and deepen your relationship with yourself. These aren't quick fixes; real transformation takes time. But these principles, once mastered, are tools you'll have for life. If you're interested in living vibrantly and loving passionately, this book will be your guide. By embracing these eight principles, we will give you the blueprint you need to turn yourself on and transform your life.

Ready to get started?

Welcome to Wonderland – down the rabbit hole we go.

Principle 1 – Assert Your Agency

By making decisions, setting and upholding boundaries, and taking command of your ship

Ever felt like things keep happening to you, like you're stuck in a real-life episode of *The Truman Show*? Where you're trying to take control but it seems like someone else is pulling the strings, and you're reacting to one thing after another? Welcome to what we call the 'No Agency Club' – membership is free, but trust us, it's not somewhere you want to stay for long.

Agency is all about taking the reins. It's about having the power to make your own decisions and act on them.[1] It's like being the captain of your own ship, navigating through the sea of life with confidence and clarity. Whether it's choosing what to have for breakfast or who you want to be in a relationship with, agency means making decisions and setting goals that reflect your values and align with who you are. It's your agency that empowers you to have more pleasurable and satisfying experiences, both in and out of the bedroom.

And yet, in a world where women often find themselves made to take a back seat in decision-making, finding your agency can feel like looking for a needle in a haystack. Whether in the boardroom or the bedroom, women face under-representation and overwhelming odds, even more so depending on factors like race, ethnicity, disabilities, gender identification and sexual orientation.[2] How's this for choice in the bedroom? Globally, only 55 per cent of married women have a say in their own healthcare, contraceptive use and the ability to say no to sex.[3] It's hard to make choices when they're being made for you. Instead of being the captain of your ship, you end up becoming a passenger.

Many of us were raised to be 'nice' and to always put other people's needs first – ever heard the old 'don't be selfish' line? Ugh, eye roll. No wonder it can feel so difficult to assert ourselves! We've all been there, going along with plans we're not into, saying 'yes' when our hearts say 'no', or consenting to sex that feels more obligatory than enjoyable. Ring any bells?

If not – we should be taking notes from you! And if so, you're not alone. Billie and I will be the first to put our hands up and say we get it, we really do. So do thousands of other women in our community, which is why we often hear them share things like:

- *'The nights when we have sex are for him, the nights when we don't are for me. I just go along with what he wants, it's easier than dealing with his defensiveness when I try to explain how I'd like to be touched differently.'*
- *'Sex feels like it's something done to me, not something I do. I'm not really part of it. It's more like a performance.'*

PRINCIPLE I – ASSERT YOUR AGENCY

- *'I don't want to be seen as a tease. We're still new and figuring things out and I really like them. I don't want them to lose interest in me.'*
- *'My partner keeps pushing me to do things I've already said no to. I know she's just joking around but it feels like she's secretly trying to wear me down.'*

Preach, sisters, we've been there too.

Here's the silver lining: asserting your agency is not only possible, it is transformative. It's essential for enjoying sex that doesn't just leave you satisfied, but makes you want to come back for more. It lays the groundwork for not only good sex, but great sex. Sex that's intimate, engaged and truly pleasurable, where you're having it not because you feel like you should, but because you genuinely want to.

And the best part? The confidence you gain in the bedroom doesn't stop there. It overflows into every other area of your life. Think about it – if you can voice what you want in bed, asking for a promotion at work suddenly doesn't seem so daunting.

This chapter is all about building the foundation to do just that. We'll cover the art of setting boundaries, the power of saying no and the importance of making decisions that genuinely feel right for you. We'll explore different types of boundaries and learn why setting a boundary isn't the same as making a request. And we'll tackle a biggie: consent – what it means, and why settling for sex you don't want is a bigger deal than you might think. By the end of this chapter, you'll be setting boundaries, honouring your body autonomy and making decisions that leave you feeling like more of a queen than Beyoncé – not just in the bedroom, but in life. Ready?

Agency case study

Straight up, having agency feels pretty dang good. It's like being the boss of your own life – calling the shots and making moves that not only feel right for you, but align with who you are and where you want to go. You're in command of the ship. But when you're lacking agency, it's a whole different story.

You feel like you're going through the motions, stuck in a loop of the same old, same old. It's like you're on autopilot, with someone else at the controls. You're watching your life happen, but you're not a part of it. To shed some light on how it can feel when your agency is taken away from you, or when you give it away, I'd like to share my own story with you.

As a heads-up, my story contains graphic content related to rape, sexual and physical violence and assault from the beginning. If that's something that might be tough for you, feel free to jump ahead to page 25.

Anna's story

It was summer. We were lying in a half-zipped sleeping bag on top of a grassy hill in the countryside – kids at my school called it 'The Look Out'. We'd come to see the stars and I'd fallen asleep.

PRINCIPLE I — ASSERT YOUR AGENCY

At first, I didn't quite know if I was dreaming. I felt the weight of his hands between my legs, his fingers delicately pulling my shorts and underwear aside, careful not to wake me. I felt confused and disoriented. I was fifteen. He was older, maybe early twenties. Even though I'd asked multiple times while we'd been hanging out over the past few months, he never revealed his age. I lay there, frozen, my brain still trying to catch up. His movements were subtle, like a spider's. Something pressed against the back of my thighs and began to push its way inside of me.

I had this abstract idea of what was happening, but I couldn't quite believe it. His breath was hot and thick against my neck, it reeked of stale cigarettes and sour cream crisps. The grip of his hand on my hip tightened, pinching my skin, and I winced. My gaze drifted upwards from the horizon as I stared at the stars and began to name constellations in my head. Ursa Major. The Big Dipper. Polaris. 'We don't have to do this if you don't want to,' he whispered as he continued to slide himself in and out of me.

I imagined myself floating in space. I was no longer connected to my body or even a part of this universe. Instead, I was a giant burning ball of hydrogen and helium, thousands of light years away. His body tensed against mine as he grunted and then collapsed against my back. He adjusted himself and pulled up his joggers. Soon after, his soft snores cut through the silence. I continued to vacantly lie there, staring blankly and feeling nothing.

My mind was completely empty save for one thought: I guess I'm not a virgin anymore.

For a long time, I kept a list. It chronicled moments in my life where my boundaries were violated or where I felt powerless. The first time I was raped was one of the earliest entries, along with some ongoing family drama. There was also the woman who followed me to school when I was sixteen and dragged me out of my car and beat me up in the parking lot. There was the taxi driver who wouldn't let me out, the men with machetes who chased me, and the guy who robbed me at gunpoint.

And the list kept growing.

There was the colleague who tried to date-rape me in university. The stranger who fingered me on my way to brunch. The peeping Tom who masturbated outside our house on Tuesdays. Oh, and the dude from Bumble. On our first date, he got naked in my living room, stood over me on the couch and slapped me in the face with his dick. Then there was the East London guy in the black Land Rover who called me a 'fucking cunt' and told me to 'get some fucking manners' for ignoring his catcalls as I walked home from the shop. I don't think he appreciated the irony when he pulled over, chased me across the street and paced outside my flat for a full seventeen minutes.

There have been many moments in my life when my agency was taken from me and my boundaries were violated. Moments that I minimized, dismissed and normalized as 'the way things are'. Unfortunately, I think that's the case for many of us – we don't realize how these moments, whether a single event or a lifetime of them, stick with us over time.

I grew up in a volatile home where I often walked on eggshells and didn't always feel safe. I also switched schools as a teenager because of being bullied by a clique who put the Plastics in Mean Girls to shame. This, combined with all these other incidents, left me feeling like my life wasn't mine for a solid thirty years. I'd worry about upsetting people, I'd struggle to say no, and I'd feel guilty about everything. Whether it was with family, friends or boyfriends, I was the 'fixer'. I was always making sure everything and everyone was okay. I'd continuously be on the lookout for something going wrong. This led to an ongoing feeling of anxiety,

PRINCIPLE 1 — ASSERT YOUR AGENCY

but it was subtle and low-level, and I could never quite pinpoint its origins. Every so often, it would flare up as a chronic uneasiness and worry, and I'd know something wasn't right, but I couldn't quite identify what it was. I couldn't put it into words, but I could feel it.

There have also been moments in my life when, through people-pleasing and failing to assert my boundaries, I unknowingly gave my agency away. Nowhere was I more of a fixer than in my romantic relationships.

Tim and I started dating when I was in my early twenties. We were together for a while, but looking back, there were so many red flags that we should have broken up sooner. A couple of years in, I discovered he'd been sending explicit photos and sexting various women, some of whom I knew. It'd been going on for months. When I called him out, he claimed it wasn't cheating because it was all online. The people-pleaser in me took over. I blamed myself. I hadn't been giving him enough attention or been a good enough partner. It was my responsibility to fix things. We were about to move in together.

Driven by my fear of hurting someone, my need to keep the peace and my inability to set boundaries, I stayed with him. Instead of asserting my agency, I gave it away. I clung to the false hope I could fix our relationship and he would change.

I spent the next two years supporting Tim's future at the expense of my own. I'd often prioritized the needs of others, but this was next-level. I failed to set boundaries, make my own decisions and assert my agency. Even when I wanted to, I couldn't bring myself to say no, because I felt bad and guilty. Despite my own best interests and my wellbeing, my people-pleasing led me to carry him in every way — emotionally, socially, financially, academically and sexually.

It was sex where I noticed it the most — and that's because sex started to hurt. I began experiencing dryness and a mild, tearing sensation during penetration. This was around the same time I caught him sexting again, but this time, I didn't confront him. Instead of feeling upset, I felt a sense of relief. Like finally I had a way out. My desire started to fade. At first, I thought I'd lost it entirely, but I realized it was only lost for him. When he was out, I'd masturbate, and I'd fantasize about different men with no issues of dryness or pain.

I came to understand that something in our relationship was broken. In its brokenness, sex became a source of tension and eventually an obligation. I didn't set boundaries because I didn't know what they were or that I needed them. Tim saw frequency of sex as a measurement of his own self-worth, and often guilted me for not initiating. He grew frustrated with my loss of desire and became passive-aggressive when he found out I was masturbating. Sometimes he did it playfully, joking that if I loved him and was committed to our relationship, I should want to have sex with him. Other times, less so. It was made out to be my duty.

And so, I complied.

I had sex I didn't want because it seemed like the path of least resistance. It meant less conflict, less pressure, less hassle. Like I said, so many red flags.

While the rest of my life moved forward, my relationship left me feeling stuck. Everything else was great; I was happy in all other aspects. And yet, when it came to sex and my romantic life, I was on autopilot. It was like I was a spectator, like sex was happening to me but I wasn't part of it. This time, unlike those other times before, my agency wasn't being taken from me. Without knowing it, I was giving it away.

PRINCIPLE 1 — ASSERT YOUR AGENCY

The science: What you need to know about asserting your agency

I realize that was a big share on my part and a lot to digest, so thank you for holding space for it – give yourself a moment to take a breath and shake it out if you need.

Now for the part where we nerd out . . .

Remember, asserting your agency is like being the captain of your ship. One of the most important things you can do as captain? Set boundaries. Boundaries are the lines you draw to map out what's acceptable and unacceptable in your relationships. This includes the most important relationship you'll ever have: the one you have with yourself. Think of boundaries as your own personal rulebook for how to become the happiest and healthiest version of you.

Boundaries: What are they and why do you need them?

Boundaries make up the foundation on which you assert your agency, because they empower you to actually exercise it. Boundaries aren't just saying 'no thanks' to others, but a 'yes please' to taking care of yourself. When you set a boundary, you don't only clarify who you're not, you also celebrate who you are and the non-negotiables that make you *you*.[4]

Boundaries cover all sorts of things, from how you

want to be treated, what you're comfortable with and how you engage with other people and things (like time, money and technology). From who you choose to hang out with, how you spend your time together and whether you split the bill, to how often you check your email or reply to your messages, boundaries help you to set expectations and assert your needs, both with others and yourself. When you've got healthy boundaries, it's like having a supercharged immune system for your mind – keeping the bad stuff out and letting the good stuff in.

There are three styles of boundaries: porous (a bit too open), rigid (a bit too closed) and flexible (just right, like Goldilocks's porridge). Now, you might recognize elements of all three boundary styles within yourself, especially across different contexts (e.g. at work, with friends, during sex, etc.). Most of us, however, will tend to associate with one type of boundary more than the other two.

POROUS BOUNDARIES: THE 'YES' PEOPLE

Those of us with porous boundaries are the 'yes' people. Obvious example? Sigh, previous versions of me – like in my relationship with Tim. Porous boundaries are 'weak' and more like soft suggestions, which means they often get overlooked. We're the ultimate people-pleasers, who find it tough to make decisions or say no, and are haunted by guilt. We end up overcommitted, overwhelmed and spread too thin. We always put others first to avoid our own fear of conflict and rejection. This

PRINCIPLE I — ASSERT YOUR AGENCY

makes deciding to put ourselves first tricky, and we can battle with anxiety and burnout. Déjà vu anyone?

We also tend to overexplain, overshare and worry about being judged as a 'bad' person. We struggle when someone's upset with us because we feel responsible for their happiness and we're not great at standing our ground. We also risk becoming co-dependent and often find ourselves becoming 'fixers' or 'saviours'. In our romantic relationships, we might be pressured or taken for granted, leaving us feeling obligated and resentful.

Examples of how porous boundaries show up during sex . . .

- Skipping foreplay even though you enjoy it
- Having sex because you think you should, not because you want to
- Finding certain positions painful, but going along with them to please a partner
- Doing a sexual act or letting yourself be touched somewhere you're not comfortable with
- Faking orgasms or performing sex

RIGID BOUNDARIES: THE 'NO' PEOPLE

Those of us with rigid boundaries are 'no' people. Our boundaries are often inflexible and more like strict rules. Once we've decided, we've decided — and that's it. Privacy and personal space are super important to us, sometimes to the extreme. We follow a code of conduct that's strict and unwavering, and we tend to see things in black-and-white and absolutes. When our boundaries are challenged, we get defensive and highly protective. In our romantic relationships, we might keep intimacy, sexual connection and opportunities for pleasure at arm's length. We have high expectations and find it tough to ask for help. We also get uncomfortable with vulnerability and openness. Instead, we spend a lot of energy keeping a safe distance, which can leave us feeling lonely and more likely to get depressed.

Examples of how rigid boundaries show up during sex . . .

- Refusing to kiss or have foreplay
- Sex being something you either have or don't
- Having lots of rules around sex (like only having sex in the dark)
- Not being open to trying new things in bed
- Keeping fantasies private and not discussing them

FLEXIBLE BOUNDARIES: THE 'YES' AND 'NO' PEOPLE

Those of us with flexible boundaries are the people who know when to say yes and when to say no. We're also at ease when other people say no to us too. Our boundaries are clear and we stand by them. We can easily adapt to different situations and consider our needs while also respecting the needs of others. We're self-aware and know our values, opinions and beliefs. We're comfortable sharing but we also appreciate privacy. That means we know when and what to share (and when and what not to). We don't feel the need to overexplain or defend our decisions. We ask for help when we need it and trust ourselves and others. We don't worry about whether our boundaries will make us less likeable because we find our sense of worth, approval and belonging from within.

Examples of how flexible boundaries show up during sex . . .

- Switching between giving and receiving during foreplay
- Enjoying cuddling or other intimate activities when not feeling up for sex itself
- Mixing up positions and checking in with each other to see what works
- Expressing and discussing sexual preferences
- Focusing on pleasure, not orgasm

Agency and your body

When it comes to having great sex, agency is like the ultimate playlist. It lets you choose the tracks that make you feel good – and switch them up depending on your mood – so you can find your own groove and have a pleasurable boogie. Without agency, the whole vibe changes. You're stuck listening to someone else's music and you're unsure about whether you'll like what comes next. This is where the connection between agency and consent comes in . . .

BOUNDARIES AND CONSENT

Two of the best peas in a pod you'll ever meet.

That's because boundaries and consent allow you to assert your agency so you can lay down the law when it comes to your body. Whether it's choosing what to wear or what type of contraception to use, guess how these decisions get made? That's right, through setting boundaries, exercising autonomy and giving or withholding consent. That's agency!

Right now, you might be thinking, 'Yeah, yeah. I know what consent is, I'm going to skip ahead.'

Don't.

Let's start by dispelling the old myth that consent is a verbal 'yes' or the absence of a 'no'. It's not. Consent is *freely* and *readily* choosing to participate in a sexual activity.* We're also talking about *all* activities, not just sex. When you give consent, it's not like a phone contract – just because you signed up once doesn't mean you're locked in. You can decide to cancel any time you want and do so without penalty. Likewise, just because you've signed up for one service doesn't mean you've signed up for them all.

Pretty straightforward, right? Agreed . . .

---

* The legal definitions of consent vary from place to place. This is a general definition that we've drawn on based on various resources, sex education platforms and advocacy organizations.

PRINCIPLE I – ASSERT YOUR AGENCY

And yet, one in two rapes against women are carried out by partners or ex-partners.[5] That, plus Billie's and my own experiences, plus the thousands of conversations we've had with other women, shows that there is (somehow) still confusion around the 'freely' and 'readily' parts.

When we talk about consent, we often focus on the obvious no-gos, like when someone is incapacitated or unconscious. But what about the times when someone feels pressured, guilt-tripped or threatened? To feel pressured or threatened is to be persuaded, influenced or intimidated into doing something, because you're worried or afraid you will be hurt or punished in some way if you don't. Most of the time, these situations happen with someone we know where it's not a case of stranger danger. Yes, you might feel like all of this sounds a little extreme, and it might not describe your experience – hopefully that's the case. But hurt and punishment can take on all sorts of different forms and it's not always what you think.

Take my relationship with Tim.

Sulking, ignoring, rejecting, criticizing, blaming – all of these can hurt. That's because hurt can be mental and emotional too. While legally my experience with Tim may not have qualified as rape, in terms of the 'freely' side of things in the informal definition, it's more blurry. There was a ton of pressure to have sex, not because I wanted to but because I felt that I was supposed to, and I was afraid of the relationship fallout that would happen if I didn't.

And then there's the 'readily' part of consent. It

often takes a back seat, especially in long-term or toxic relationships. Ever heard (or said) things like 'It's easier to say yes' or 'I don't want to lead them on'? That's what we're talking about. The formal term for this is 'sexual compliance'. It's when you say yes to sex not because you're into it, but because you want more intimacy, to make your partner happy or to keep the peace.[6] Ring any bells?

Sigh. This is how I spent years in some of my previous relationships. Billie's done it too, as you'll hear from her later. And even though we know better, it's *still* something we sometimes do. Old habits die hard, right?

But here's the kicker: every time you comply with sex because you think it'll make your partner happy, you're trading in your own happiness instead.[7] Sex becomes this sort of self-sacrifice, where you put someone else's needs above your own. It's people-pleasing, but the sex edit. You're not having sex because you want to, but because you think you should. Sure, it might not seem like a big deal in the moment, but every time you make the decision to have unwanted sex, you're giving away a tiny piece of your agency (and yourself too). Think of yourself as a puzzle – eventually all those missing pieces add up and you're left with a picture that's incomplete.

It doesn't have to be like this though. There are many ways we can assert our agency, starting with making healthy decisions and having healthy boundaries, both in and out of the bedroom.

PRINCIPLE 1 — ASSERT YOUR AGENCY

Examples of healthy boundaries

Setting healthy boundaries is like drawing a personal map of where you end and others begin. It's about making decisions about what's acceptable to you and what's not, and letting everyone know the rules of your space. Here are some examples . . .

EMOTIONAL: BOUNDARIES RELATED TO FEELINGS

- **With partners:** 'I'd like us to spend some quality time together outside of the house. I've planned a fun date for us this Saturday.'
- **With friends:** 'It sounds like you're going through a rough patch and I'm not the best person to support. Have you thought about therapy?'
- **With family:** 'I get that family stuff is important, but I'm not going to talk about getting married or having kids. I'd appreciate it if you stopped asking.'

PHYSICAL: BOUNDARIES RELATED TO BODIES AND PHYSICAL SPACE

- **With yourself:** 'I'm not big on hugging strangers. I'm sticking to handshakes from now on.'

- **With family:** 'As a heads-up, my diet is [X]. Please don't give me a rough time about it and you don't have to whip up anything special – I can bring my own food.'
- **With work:** 'Desk time is work time for me. If you want to chat, I'm happy to share my calendar with you and we can schedule a catch-up.'

SEXUAL: BOUNDARIES RELATED TO SEX

- **With yourself:** 'If I'm not feeling like sex, I'll let my partner know and set time aside for us to have a chat about what I need to get in the mood.'
- **With a partner:** 'I respect that your desire's been low. Touch is important to me and I'd like us to brainstorm how we can meet each other's needs halfway.'
- **With work:** 'The sex jokes aren't cool, they make me uncomfortable. I'm going to ignore them so we can keep it professional.'

TEMPORAL: BOUNDARIES RELATED TO TIME

- **With a partner:** 'You're a night owl and I'm an early bird. I'm hitting the hay now so I can wake up early.'
- **With friends:** 'Thank you for the invite. I can't make it but have a blast.'

PRINCIPLE I — ASSERT YOUR AGENCY

- **With work:** 'I'm all for getting this project done, but my workday ends at five. I'll pick this back up first-thing when I get in in the morning.'

INTELLECTUAL: BOUNDARIES RELATED TO THOUGHTS, IDEAS AND OPINIONS

- **With a partner:** 'I need some time to sit with things. I'll sync up with you tomorrow.'
- **With friends:** 'I'm not into talking about [name] when they're not here. How's the rest of your week going?'
- **With family:** 'We're on different pages here and that's okay. Let's chat about something else, yeah?'

MATERIAL: BOUNDARIES RELATED TO THINGS (LIKE MONEY, BELONGINGS, TECHNOLOGY)

- **With yourself:** 'My bedtime's been creeping because I've been on my phone before bed. Time to get an alarm clock so I don't sleep with my phone next to me.'
- **With a partner:** 'Solo play is important to me. When I do this, I'm going to use my vibrator and read erotica.'
- **With friends:** 'When we go out, let's split the bill. I'll cover my half, you cover yours.'

Asserting agency in real life

In a world that's constantly telling us how to live, asserting our agency is like giving ourselves permission to be the authors of our own story. For Billie and I, asserting our agency has helped us step into our own power so we're not going through the motions on autopilot – be it with sex, relationships or life – and we're actively deciding our future. Asserting your agency is about embracing who you are and what you want, and making choices that align with who you are from the inside out. Here's what that looked like for me . . .

When I sat down to write this share, I wasn't sure where to begin. I think that's because deconstructing and reconstructing ourselves is about as straightforward as following an IKEA manual – it ain't always easy. It's taken me years to learn how to assert my agency, and I still catch myself getting it wrong. Boundary-wise, I also did a hard swing from porous to rigid and back again, before I finally managed to land on flexible. Turns out ditching a lifetime of people-pleasing is hard work. Who knew?

To give you a glimpse of what this has looked like in real life, let's catch up on how I've been getting better at asserting my agency.

Cool?

Cool.

Breaking up with Tim left me feeling relief, freedom and joy. Like taking your bra off after a long day and finally being able to breathe. I used to get a lot of nightmares – no surprise there, my subconscious was a hot mess back in the day. Nowadays, they're

PRINCIPLE 1 — ASSERT YOUR AGENCY

rare, but when they do pop up, it's always one or two of my exes in the lead role.

Why, you ask?

Here's my take: repeatedly having sex because I felt like I should, not because I wanted to, left a mark. It fundamentally changed the nature of my relationships and how I perceived my partners at the time, even though it was me who was complying. Every time I did, I considered them as a sort of 'villain', both in my head and in bed. The more I acted out of obligation or duty, the more I lost my desire – not for sex, but for sex with them. Over time, more resentment built, and I couldn't come back from it.

Now, having spent years working to reclaim my agency both in and out of the bedroom, there's no way in hell I'm letting go of it again. Let me tell you, I'm holding on to it tighter than two sea otters holding hands.

Fast-forward to how I'm asserting my agency in the present . . .

While writing this chapter, I had to revisit some not-so-great sexual experiences, which didn't exactly put me in the mood for sex. Not understanding this, there were a few times during this period when my current partner, Luke, tried to initiate.

Old me would have thought: 'Ugh, I don't want to but I feel like I should and I feel bad saying no, so okay, fine. Let's get it over with.' And I would have gone along with it, telling myself it was easier that way.

But hello, Anna 2.0.

New me set boundaries. One with myself, to stop being sexually compliant. And another with Luke – I communicated 'no' to sex but that I was open to other sexy activities. Without going into too much pillow talk, it was great and we both had fun.

The second time, it was pretty similar – nothing to report.

The third time though, the old people-pleaser in me started creeping back in. I felt guilty, and all the 'shoulds' came flooding back. But instead of brushing her aside, I sat with her for a moment. I realized I hadn't been fully upfront with Luke about why I was feeling less frisky, which wasn't fair to him. So, instead of suggesting other types of sexy play, we had a heart-to-heart. I shared what was going on and we brainstormed ways to meet his needs and keep our intimacy alive without me feeling pressured to have sex.

I also made the decision to keep my work life and relationship life separate while working on this chapter. I set a boundary to take solo walks to decompress after work, and booked some therapy sessions to ensure I had the right support system in place.

What's been a game changer for me is to understand the difference between setting a boundary and making a request. In the early days, I didn't know how to set them, and got frustrated when other people didn't respect my 'boundaries'. I eventually learned from listening to therapists like Nedra Glover Tawwab and clinical psychologists like Becky Kennedy that a boundary is a line you draw that says, 'This is okay, and this isn't' — it's something you do, and it doesn't require the other person to do anything.[8]

This was a revelation for me. I'd 100 per cent been making requests, not setting boundaries. The prime example was with condoms. When I moved to the UK, I was shocked by how many guys thought they weren't necessary because I had an IUD. I'd ask them to wear one, and I reckon 75 per cent of them huffed and puffed about whether it was necessary and complained about how it didn't feel as good. Soz, dude, neither does chlamydia. It would become this awkward negotiation where I'd end up justifying and defending myself. So, I changed tactics. Instead of making

PRINCIPLE I – ASSERT YOUR AGENCY

a request in the moment, I set a boundary ahead of time and earlier in the date: 'I won't have sex without a condom.' It was an absolute game changer – no more haggling, no more explaining, just an easy and enjoyable good time.

The other way I've been working on asserting my agency is to make decisions rather than putting them off. That was something I used to do all the time, like when I delayed the decision to break up way back when. I call it 'decision drift'. It's where we avoid making the decisions we know we need to make now, which leaves them to drift along downstream, where we eventually catch up with them later. So, I started making small decisions that were low-risk. Becoming the captain of my own ship and all that.

When friends asked me, 'Where do you want to meet?', rather than saying, 'Wherever's best for you', I'd decide. Gradually, the small decisions got bigger. During sex, when partners would ask me, 'What do you want?', I'd tell them more kissing, a slower pace and longer foreplay. I stopped complying and started consenting and communicating, which led to enthusiastic heck yeses. As for the big decisions, I made sure to set aside time to review them every 1–2 weeks using the Eisenhower Matrix (a tool we've got for you on p. 46). Instead of avoiding my decisions, I'd organize them and prioritize where to start. This helped me to feel more in command of my life – my agency was making a comeback, one decision at a time.

So, no more sitting on the sidelines, observing your journey as a passer-by. It's up to you to create your map and plot your course across all aspects of your life.

The unfortunate reality is that sometimes we don't have a choice; sometimes our ability to choose is taken from us or didn't even exist to begin with. For better and worse there are so many things that are outside of our control. What *is* within our control though, is how we choose to show up for ourselves and others. If there's one thing we want you to take away from this chapter, it's that asserting your agency matters. By understanding your boundary type, learning how to set them and getting better at making decisions – whether they're big or small – you can find your power and take command of that all-important ship, both in and out of the bedroom.

In practice: Here's how to assert your agency

Tool #1: Identify your boundary style and score your boundary types

Before we get into the nitty-gritty of setting and sticking to your boundaries, let's figure out what kinds of boundaries you're working with right now. Since we know you're interested in sex, we'll start by looking at your boundaries in the bedroom. Check out the statements below and mark any that feel true for you.

Porous

- __ I often worry about being good in bed and if my partner is satisfied.
- __ I tend to say yes to sex, even when I'm not in the mood.

PRINCIPLE 1 – ASSERT YOUR AGENCY

___ I sometimes feel like my willingness to accommodate my partner's needs is taken for granted.
___ I don't feel confident expressing my desires or saying no to things I'm not comfortable with.
___ I prioritize others' needs and wants, often at the expense of my own wellbeing.

Rigid

___ I like to keep my desires private and often keep my sexual partner(s)* at a distance.
___ I prefer not to show vulnerability or emotions during intimate moments.
___ I have lots of rules around sex and I prefer to have it in the way that I want.
___ I am uncomfortable with unexpected changes or spontaneity in my sexual encounters.
___ I am strict about my personal space during sex and how and when I like to be touched.

Flexible

___ I feel confident expressing my sexual desires and saying yes or no to sex without guilt.
___ I am comfortable finding a balance in activities that satisfy both my partner and me.

---

* Throughout the book we use the word 'partner' to refer to a partner, and multiple partners for those of you who are dating more casually or in consensual non-monogamous relationships.

___ I can respectfully communicate what I consider to be acceptable and unacceptable behaviour.
___ I am open to my partner's needs and can adjust my boundaries when it feels right to do so.
___ I don't take it personally or get defensive when my partner says no to certain activities.

As you go through the statements and mark the ones that feel true for you, think about which category you're ticking most often. This will give you a good sense of your main boundary style. It's normal to have checks in more than one category because your boundary style can change depending on the situation.

SCORE YOUR BOUNDARY TYPES

After you've marked your statements, take a moment to think about how these different boundary styles show up in your life. Keep in mind that just as there are different boundary styles (porous, rigid and flexible), there are also different types of boundaries, like the ones we explored on pp. 33–35. Your boundary style is how you set and maintain boundaries, whereas boundary types are the 'categories' of boundaries you are setting.

The following list can help you to reflect on how comfortable you are with setting and sticking to different boundary types, as well as how you respect the boundary types set by others. Give each type a score from 1 to 5, where 1 means it's not a strong suit and 5 means you've got it down. This will help you identify

PRINCIPLE I — ASSERT YOUR AGENCY

which types of boundaries you might want to focus on improving first.

- __ **Sexual boundaries:** I set and uphold boundaries related to sex and sexual behaviours and I respect those of others.
- __ **Emotional boundaries:** I set and uphold boundaries related to my feelings and emotions and I respect those of others.
- __ **Physical boundaries:** I set and uphold boundaries related to my body, non-sexual touch and physical space and I respect those of others.
- __ **Temporal boundaries:** I set and uphold boundaries related to my time, how I spend it and what I do with it, and I respect those of others.
- __ **Intellectual boundaries:** I set and uphold boundaries related to my thoughts, ideas and opinions, and I respect those of others.
- __ **Material boundaries:** I set and uphold boundaries related to my belongings, money and technology and I respect those of others.

Tool #2: Choose a boundary type and set three boundaries

Now that you have your scores, pick a boundary type from the previous list that stands out to you. Challenge yourself to set three boundaries related to this type. These could be boundaries with yourself, your partner, friends, family or even at work. It's not just about stating your boundaries, it's also about sticking to them. Some people will respect your boundaries, while others might not, and that's okay. You're responsible for yourself, and they're responsible for themselves.

Here's a general **script** for you to follow, to help you with some examples of what it might look like in a conversation. Depending on the context, obviously you can tweak it:

> *[Description of a specific situation in which difficult behaviour occurred]* – when *[specific behaviour that happened]* I felt *[emotion]*. It's important for me to have a *[type of boundary]* in place because it helps me *[reason for boundary]*. Moving forward, I'm going to *[boundary you are setting]*. If *[specific behaviour]* happens again, I will *[action you are going to take to uphold your boundary]*. Thank you for understanding.

Full disclosure, **this script is going to feel formal, and that's okay**. It's kind of the point – it makes it easier to follow and helps you avoid overexplaining yourself or accidentally criticizing the other person.

Here are some examples:

- 'Hey, remember last Tuesday at dinner with our friends when I tried to give you a kiss, but you turned away? I felt embarrassed and rejected in the moment. Talking about physical boundaries is important to me because it helps me feel secure and understand differences we might have around what we're comfortable doing

PRINCIPLE 1 — ASSERT YOUR AGENCY

in public. I'd like us to explore this together, so I'm setting aside some time for us to chat it through. If you don't want to have this conversation, I'll need to think about how else to make this relationship work for me.'
- 'When we woke up on Saturday morning, I noticed we were both on our phones. Because we don't get to sleep in and have a cuddle during the week, I felt bummed out about not making the most of it. It's important for me to have that quality time together without distractions because it helps me feel connected to you and intimate. This weekend, I'm going to hold off on checking my phone when I wake up and I'd love it if you'd do that too. Otherwise, I think we should leave our phones in the other room before bed.'
- 'When we had sex yesterday, you didn't go down on me and I felt disappointed because I enjoy it when you do. I also felt a little self-conscious and unattractive because it's been a while since you last did it. It's important to me that you don't do anything you don't want to in bed, while also honouring my needs. I'm keen to experiment with taking turns giving and receiving before we have sex. If that's not something you're up for then I'd appreciate it if you could help me understand why.'

Tool #3: Use the Eisenhower Matrix to help make decisions

The Eisenhower Matrix is a tool that both Billie and I swear by when it comes to sorting out our decisions (as well as to-do lists). It's like having a personal assistant for your brain, helping you figure out what decisions need your attention ASAP and what can take a back seat. For this exercise you'll need somewhere to write a list, as well as a pen or pencil and a piece of paper to draw on.

Here are your step-by-step instructions:

1. **Make a list:** In a notebook or on your phone, jot down all the decisions you need to make or tasks you've got on your plate.
2. **Sketch it out:** Now, grab a piece of paper and draw a big square or download the template from www.turnyourselfon.co. If drawing, split your square into four smaller squares. Above the top two squares, write 'Urgent' and 'Not Urgent', and next to the left two squares, write 'Important' and 'Not Important'.
3. **Sort it out:** Place each decision or task in one of the four boxes . . .
    a. **Top left:** Important and Urgent (these are your top priorities).
    b. **Top right:** Important but Not Urgent (plan a time to tackle these – they're important, but there's no rush).

PRINCIPLE I — ASSERT YOUR AGENCY

   c. **Bottom left:** Not Important but Urgent (if you can, pass these off to someone else – they need to get actioned, but not necessarily by you).
   d. **Bottom right:** Not Important and Not Urgent (these are your lowest priority – you can either put them off for later or ditch them altogether).
4. **Get to work:** Start with the 'Important and Urgent' decisions or tasks and then schedule the 'Important but Not Urgent' ones for later. Find someone to take care of the 'Not Important but Urgent' decisions or tasks and think about whether you really need to do the 'Not Important and Not Urgent' ones at all.
5. **Keep it fresh:** Regularly check in on your list to see if anything's changed in terms of importance or urgency.

Look back to look forward

Take 1–2 minutes to reflect and answer the following questions:

1. How am I asserting my agency well?
2. How am I not asserting my agency well?
3. What's one action I'm going to start, stop or continue NOW to assert my agency in my life?

TURN YOURSELF ON

> If you'd like to dive deeper, we've hooked you up with some great resources and downloadable templates at www.turnyourselfon.co.

Cement your learnings

- **Agency:** It's like being the captain of your own ship. You're in charge of your life and get to shape how it unfolds. When you've got agency, you're more likely to feel happy and healthy, both in and out of the bedroom.
- **Boundaries:** These are the lines you draw to define what's cool and what's not cool for you, both with yourself and others. There are three types:
  - **Porous boundaries:** Too open, letting in stuff that shouldn't get in.
  - **Rigid boundaries:** Too closed, keeping out stuff that might be good.
  - **Flexible boundaries:** Just right, letting in the good stuff and keeping out the bad.
- **Asserting agency with boundaries:** Boundaries are your toolkit for asserting agency. They can be emotional, physical, sexual, temporal, intellectual or material. And remember, setting a boundary is different from making a request – it's about what *you* do, not what someone else needs to do.

PRINCIPLE I – ASSERT YOUR AGENCY

- **Consent and body autonomy:** This is a super-important type of boundary, especially when it comes to sex. It's about freely and readily choosing to participate in sexual activity and having autonomy over what happens to your body. If it's not freely and readily given, it's not consent.
- **Keeping your agency strong:** Agency isn't something you have, it's a skill you build. You strengthen it by setting and sticking to your boundaries, making decisions and taking command of your ship.

Bonus reads

- Paul Napper, PsyD, and Anthony Rao, PhD, *The Power of Agency: The 7 Principles to Conquer Obstacles, Make Effective Decisions & Create a Life on Your Own Terms*
- Nedra Glover Tawwab, *Set Boundaries, Find Peace: A Guide to Reclaiming Yourself*
- Dr Henry Cloud and Dr John Townsend, *Boundaries: When to Say Yes, How to Say No to Take Control of Your Life*
- Daniel Kahneman, *Thinking Fast and Slow*
- Stephanie Foo, *What My Bones Know: A Memoir of Healing from Complex Trauma*
- Resmaa Menakem, *My Grandmother's Hands: Racialized Trauma and the Pathway to Mending Our Hearts and Bodies*

- Richard Schwartz, PhD, *No Bad Parts: Healing Trauma and Restoring Wholeness with the Internal Family Systems Model*
- Roxane Gay, *Not That Bad: Dispatches from Rape Culture*
- Laura Bates, *Men Who Hate Women: From Incels to Pick Up Artists: The Truth About Extreme Misogyny and How It Affects Us All*

Principle 2 – Balance Your Power

*By ditching the idea of 'power over'
and strengthening your feeling of
'power to' and 'power with'*

Power. It's a big topic and a hot one – since, well, forever. From Plato and Aristotle through Machiavelli and Hobbes, there's a lot of philosophizing going on, so let's keep it simple. Power is your ability to influence another person or situation, while also having the ability not to be influenced in return.[1] Whether we admit it or not, power plays a role in every relationship we have. When it's balanced in our relationships, power can be the force that nurtures and uplifts us, while keeping things on an even keel. It's sort of like a secret ingredient that lets us treat each other as equals and ensure that respect is flowing both ways.

Here's the kicker though: when power becomes imbalanced, our relationships don't feel so good and things can feel a bit off. It doesn't matter if you're the one holding the reins or if someone else is calling the shots, imbalances in power can create tension, drive resentment and wreck relationships.

When it comes to power imbalances and sex, the

numbers aren't pretty. In the UK, one in ten women report having had sex against their will – in other words, someone else asserted power over them.[2] Sixty-one per cent of the time the person responsible was a current or former partner, a family member or a friend. Unfortunately, unlike committed same-sex relationships where the power balance is more even, there's a common imbalance in heterosexual relationships, with the power being held mostly by men. This can have not-so-great consequences in terms of how different genders experience sex.[3]

Unsurprisingly, this power imbalance is reversed when it comes to household decision-making. A study by the Pew Research Center, which looked into the lives of 1,260 American couples, found that women called the shots 43 per cent of the time. This was followed by decisions being made equally 31 per cent of the time, and 26 per cent of the time being made by men.[4] That's to say, finding a balance of power in our relationships matters – and yet, navigating power can sometimes feel messy. That's because it's not always the case that one person in the relationship holds all the power all of the time.

In this chapter, we're going to explore the concept of power – what it is and what it's not. We'll look at three different ways power can affect your relationships – 'power over', 'power to' and 'power with' – and how you can balance it more evenly. Plus, we'll check out some behaviours – the good, the bad and the ugly – that can help you figure out if the power dynamic in your relationships is healthy or heading for trouble. Getting

PRINCIPLE 2 — BALANCE YOUR POWER

a grip on the different types of power and how they can show up in your relationships can give you a better picture of what a good power balance looks like. The more you learn about your own personal power and how to share power with others, the more able you'll be to create happier and healthier relationships overall.

Power case study

Whether it's in the bedroom or the boardroom, the dance between sex and power can show up anywhere. The first type of power we're going to explore — and one you might already know a thing or two about — is called 'power over'. To give you a feel for what 'power over' looks like in relationships, Billie has offered to get vulnerable and share her story of sexual assault. Through her words, you'll get a real sense of how power can be misused and abused in both a professional and a sexual context.

Just a heads-up, this story does contain graphic content related to sexual assault at work. If that's something that might be tough for you, feel free to jump ahead to page 58.

Billie's story

When I was in my mid-twenties, I was offered a junior sales role at a company in the City of London. It was an amazing opportunity to start building my career, and I felt like my future was beginning to take shape. During one of my training days, Robert, a senior team member, offered to mentor me. Even though I'd just started, we got on well and had a nice dynamic. As the only woman on the team and being 30–40 years younger than everyone else, I was both nervous and excited to hold my own. Later that week, Robert and I had our first mentoring session in the boardroom. We talked about the company's expectations, navigating office politics, and how he wanted to help me advance my career. Overall, it was a pretty standard session and I felt good about it. I was grateful to him for volunteering his time and for helping me step into my new role.

Then came our second meeting. I'd booked a meeting room but Robert decided at the last minute that we should go to a bar. He told me that we'd catch up one-to-one first, and then join the rest of the team elsewhere for weekly drinks. The bar itself was empty and quiet. Robert suggested we sit at the back so we wouldn't be overheard discussing clients or anything confidential. He chose a corner table that was behind a pillar and hidden from view.

As soon as we sat down, Robert asked me what I wanted to drink and I told him I'd like a green tea. Laughing, he replied, 'No, no. Come on now. Let's have a drink,' as he ordered two double gin and tonics and a shot of tequila for himself.

We got to chatting and immediately he directed our conversation towards personal things. Without being rude, I tried to steer it back to work but he ignored me. Within the first half an hour, he knocked back three double G&Ts and a couple of shots. I'd barely touched my first drink and yet he continued to order me more without asking. The drunker he got, the more intrusive the conversation became. I felt uneasy and uncertain but I wasn't sure what to do. I told myself not to read into it. That he was in his

PRINCIPLE 2 – BALANCE YOUR POWER

sixties and this was just banter and part of the culture. Then he started talking about his wife.

Louise also worked at our office and was senior to me, albeit in a different team. He began to share intimate details of their marriage and how much he liked sex. 'What is happening right now?' I thought to myself. He took another swig of his drink and brushed his hand against my knee under the table. I froze. Looking at me, Robert purred, 'I love to lick her out. I love to lick all women out. I love the taste of their pussies and how it feels when I put my tongue inside of them.' My throat went dry. I could feel the rapid thump-thump-thump of my heart in my chest. All I could think about was how hot and clammy his hand was against my skin as he continued to stroke my knee.

'Robert, that's really inappropriate.'

'No, come on, it's not inappropriate,' he chided. 'We're just having a drink and getting to know each other. We're sharing what we enjoy, don't be so prudish.' More knee stroking and another swig of gin. 'Go on, tell me. What do you like, Billie?' He pushed his chair closer, positioning himself beside me.

My breath quickened and my muscles tensed. I suddenly became aware of how tall and big he was, how much his body towered over my own.

'I really don't feel comfortable discussing this.'

'Why?' He laughed and rolled his eyes. 'Isn't your generation supposed to be sexually liberated? All I'm saying is that I like giving women head and I'm very good at it. Don't you like getting licked out?' He squeezed my knee a little harder.

'Robert, this conversation feels like it's getting a bit silly.' I stood up to flag the server, but he grabbed me by the waist and pulled me down onto his lap. I panicked. My mind was racing as

I tried to make sense of what was happening and to figure out what to do. 'Come on, Robert, let's go somewhere else.'

His stroke moved from the top of my knee to the inside of my leg. Frantically, I managed to squirm loose and wave down our server for the bill.

Unsure what would happen when we left, as Robert was settling up I quickly texted a friend who I knew was out for dinner round the corner. I told him that I needed help and to come now. Robert moved to leave, but was so drunk he nearly fell over. He immediately put his arm around my shoulders, crushing me under his weight. As we stumbled between the tables, he kept talking about women's pussies and I could feel his breath, wet and hot against my neck. Once on the street, he pushed me against the wall and pinned me with his arms. He was so strong. Fuck, fuck, fuck. This couldn't actually be happening.

I managed to duck under one of his arms, but as I did he grabbed my hand and spun me around, pinning me once more between the wall and his weight. His eyes, glazed and red, scanned my body up and down. He licked his lips and then started to kiss me. I froze, my entire body rigid. I remember the taste of gin as he forced his tongue into my mouth and down my throat. I pulled my head away in disgust. He leaned back and started laughing.

'Billie?' I heard my friend call from down the street. Robert stepped back and grabbed my hand, pulling me in the opposite direction.

'Let's go,' he said.

'No, no, that's my boyfriend,' I lied. 'I'm going to stay.' I could hardly speak; I was shaking so much. I felt like I was about to be sick.

My friend managed to get Robert in a cab and sent him home. About an hour later, I got a text. Robert wanted to let

PRINCIPLE 2 — BALANCE YOUR POWER

me know he'd gotten home safe and asked if I could come over and put him to bed. I didn't register what had happened, I just sort of . . . detached. I told myself that he was really drunk and probably didn't mean it, that I shouldn't make it into a big deal.

I took the next day off work. I didn't quite know how to face him. He sent another message, this time commenting about how funny last night was, that he'd been so drunk and he couldn't wait for our next mentoring session. My stomach churned.

Later that week, I was walking back to my desk. Robert was in a meeting with a bunch of the senior execs.

'Oi, yellow dress!' he shouted across the office at me. 'Your pins look absolutely amazing!' He turned to the rest of the men and added, 'Don't her legs look great?' They all laughed and nodded.

I kept my head up and walked straight to the bathroom, where I started to cry. I not only felt undermined but humiliated. My mind was racing. 'This is because of me. I'm obviously inviting this behaviour. I can't tell anyone because it's my fault. It was just a bit of banter anyways. I just need to put my head down.' Immediately after work, I bought two long-sleeved black dresses, black trousers, a black turtleneck, thick black tights and a pair of black trainers. As someone who was always playful and charismatic, I now made it my mission to dull my personality. I avoided talking to my male colleagues. I stopped making jokes and I forbade myself from laughing. I forced myself to become small, insignificant and unnoticeable.

In the months that followed, I fell into a deep depression. My performance at work suffered, and even though I was surrounded by people, I felt isolated and alone. I struggled to build workplace relationships because I was afraid of myself and scared of my sexuality and that it would be misunderstood. Everything took effort, and I'd often find myself crying for no reason. My body was foreign, like it was no longer mine. In the moments between apathy and numbness, I felt angry. Not at Robert, but at myself for letting this happen and for not doing more to fight back. I knew power was a thing, but I didn't really understand how it showed up in life or in my relationships. I also didn't know about all the various forms the abuse of power could take. All I knew was that something bad had happened and I was responsible.

The science: What you need to know about power

Power dynamics in relationships

To help you navigate the ways power plays out in your relationships – both in your sex life and broader life too – we're going to break down three different types of power. These are: 'power over', 'power to' and 'power with'.

POWER OVER

'Power over' is when one person holds the reins. It's asymmetrical, and typically comes with coercive, controlling and manipulative behaviours. Picture someone putting pressure on another person to do something, or using guilt, shame or fear to steer someone's choices or actions. Think Robert.

'Power over' is about establishing dominance, but it

PRINCIPLE 2 — BALANCE YOUR POWER

doesn't always show up as violence or obvious attacks.[5] Sometimes it's glaring, as in Billie's sexual assault. Other times, it's sneakier, like giving someone the silent treatment or even disguising itself as playful banter or teasing. Sadly, not all nice people are always as nice as they seem.

Unsurprisingly, privilege is also a huge factor when it comes to people having power over others. Many of us juggle multiple overlapping identities, shaped by things like our gender, race, sexual orientation, class and disabilities. These identities intersect and create different experiences of privilege and power. For instance, women with disabilities in the UK are nearly twice as likely to face sexual assault as those without.[6] Over in the US, a staggering 56 per cent of Indigenous women have experienced sexual violence.[7] And these numbers can be even more daunting, as many women of colour don't report instances of assault due to issues like inadequate service provision, institutional racism and police brutality.[8,9] It goes without saying that people like Robert hold a lot of privilege – which, in turn, allows them to assume power over others. It also goes without saying that while someone might have those privileges, which are out of their control, it's their choice to use their privilege to gain power over others.

From the sheets to the streets, 'power over' plays a huge role in shaping our day-to-day lives. It might even be the only way that you had considered people having power until now, and that's okay. The good news is – that's not the case.

POWER TO

The second type of power is all about tapping into your inner personal power and believing in yourself, getting things done on your own, maintaining your agency and being resilient when things get tough. It's a knack for self-regulating and keeping your cool, understanding and sharing your feelings, and staying true to your voice while respecting the voices of others.[10]

In the bedroom, 'power to' shows up in actions like standing up for your intimate needs, asserting your agency and expressing yourself sexually. Unlike 'power over', which is having power over someone else, 'power to' is about having power over yourself. It's about having the freedom to choose and make things happen – it's being the boss of yourself. Both in and out of the bedroom, your 'power to' is the bedrock of who you are and everything you do. After all, if you don't have your own power, it's tough to have any power at all.

POWER WITH

The third type of power is the classic 'we' power that you share with someone else or a group of other people. 'Power with' is all about teamwork, collaboration and splitting the load.[11] When it comes to sex and intimacy, it's about you and your partner taking responsibility and being dedicated to shaping your relationship and its overall wellbeing.[12] 'Power with' is built on having common goals, collective input and striving towards a shared mission. This kind of power comes from being

PRINCIPLE 2 – BALANCE YOUR POWER

in sync with others and creating situations where relationships are more balanced.

In the bedroom, 'power with' shows up as honouring consent, focusing on mutual pleasure and making decisions together. Outside the bedroom, it's about respect, connection and fixing things when they go wrong. Together, 'power to' and 'power with' symbolize both personal and relationship empowerment and are kind of like the kryptonite to 'power over'. When put to good use, these behaviours can be cooperative, generative and reciprocal.

Now that you've got an outline of the three different types of relationship power, it's helpful to look at some examples of behaviours that go along with them.

The red flags: Abusive 'power over' behaviours

First up, let's talk about red flags. These are 'power over' behaviours that not only show there's a power imbalance but also that there's an abuse of power. These are never okay, and are clear signs that a relationship is not healthy.

- **Physical:** Using physical force, violence or unwanted contact to hurt someone or make them feel physically unsafe. Examples are hitting, throwing things, driving dangerously and preventing you from entering/leaving spaces.
- **Sexual:** Forcing, pressuring or coercing someone into sex or sexual acts that they're not

comfortable with. Doing the old circle back here to body autonomy and the whole 'freely' and 'readily' parts of consent (see p. 30).
- **Psychological/emotional:** Using non-physical behaviours to harm someone's mental and emotional wellbeing by controlling and manipulating them. This can look like insulting, accusing, humiliating, isolating, threatening or gaslighting.
- **Stalking:** Repeatedly following, watching or harassing someone, and making them scared for their safety. It looks like showing up uninvited at places where they spend time, following them around or using things like GPS or 'Find My Location' to track them.
- **Digital:** Using technology – like social media, email or texts – to control, harass and/or monitor someone. Examples include trolling, catfishing, sending unwanted messages, recording without consent or snooping through private messages or search history.
- **Financial:** Controlling or manipulating someone's access to money or work. It could be things like limiting access to resources, hiding financial information, using someone's money or credit without consent, creating debt in their name or sabotaging their employment and career opportunities.

Despite being abusive behaviours, many of us tend to downplay these, or think of them as 'the way things are'. In her book *Men Who Hate Women*, journalist Laura Bates points out: 'Misogyny and violence against women are so widespread and so normalized, it is difficult for us to consider these things "extreme" or "radical", because they are simply not out of the ordinary . . . [they are] already part of the wallpaper.'[13]

But just because we've gotten used to these behaviours, it doesn't mean they're normal. And just because someone might not realize they're being abusive and their actions don't seem 'violent', it doesn't make them any less real. Even if a behaviour seems 'playful', 'affectionate' or 'flirtatious', if the intention is to pressure or manipulate someone into doing something they don't want to do – i.e. asserting power *over* them – it's a no-go.

AN EXTRA NOTE ON GASLIGHTING: WHAT IT IS AND WHY IT'S TRICKY TO CATCH

There's a specific 'power over' behaviour that Billie and I want to highlight because it can be super sneaky: gaslighting. The term 'gaslighting' comes from a 1930s British play called *Gas Light* by Patrick Hamilton, which was made into a film in 1940. Hamilton's play is set in the 1880s and focuses on Bella Manningham, who is abused by her husband, Jack. To control and break Bella, Jack starts messing with her environment – like dimming the gas lights in their house – and then denies that anything has changed. This makes Bella doubt herself and her sanity, and ultimately, Jack drives her insane.

Gaslighting is a form of psychological and emotional abuse that's incredibly effective at making someone 'question their own feelings, instincts, and sanity'.[14] And here's a key point: **gaslighting is an ongoing process rather than a one-off event.**[15]

Over time, it erodes someone's trust in themselves, which makes them more likely to stay in a relationship and in an abusive cycle. Common gaslighting tactics include:

- **Withholding: acting like they don't understand or refusing to listen.** For example, saying things like 'You're not making sense' or 'I don't have to listen to this'.
- **Countering: challenging your memory of events.** Examples: 'You're making that up'; 'I was there, that's not what happened'.
- **Diverting: shifting focus away from their behaviour.** Examples: 'I'm not the problem here'; 'You're the one with issues'.
- **Minimizing: treating your concerns and feelings as unimportant.** Examples: 'It was just a joke'; 'You're overreacting, don't be so sensitive'.
- **Denying: pretending to forget or denying having said or done something.** Examples: 'I don't know what you're talking about'; 'I never said that'.
- **Projecting: accusing you of behaviours they themselves are exhibiting.** Examples: 'You're the one getting upset, not me'; 'You're always trying to control me'.

PRINCIPLE 2 — BALANCE YOUR POWER

- **Twisting: distorting your words or actions to make you doubt yourself.** Examples: 'You're taking it out of context'; 'You know I didn't mean it like that'.

Whether it's gaslighting or any other red flag behaviour, if you're on the receiving end, know that these behaviours are not okay, that you're not alone and there are options for help. While breaking these cycles is beyond the scope of this book, we've included some resources at the end of the chapter that can offer guidance and support (see p. 89).

Likewise, if you recognize yourself as someone who exhibits abusive or red flag behaviours, it's important to take responsibility for your actions and hold yourself accountable. The first step is to acknowledge them and recognize that they can negatively impact and harm others. The second step is to get professional support so you can address the root causes of your behaviours and develop healthier ways of expressing yourself and relating to people. The resources we've included at the end of this chapter are for you too.

The amber flags: Common but destructive if left unchecked

Alright, we've tackled the red flag behaviours, now let's get to know some amber ones: criticism, defensiveness, contempt and stonewalling. In his book with Nan Silver, *The Seven Principles for Making Marriage Work*, couples' researcher and therapist Dr John Gottman dubs them 'the Four Horsemen of the Relationship Apocalypse'.[16] That's because, even though these behaviours are super common, if they're not kept in check, they're the ones most likely to wreck a relationship. How often they pop up (or not) in your relationship(s) plays a big role in shaping its overall stability, longevity and health.[17]

#1 CRITICISM

First up is criticism. This is when we go after another person's character and sense of self, instead of addressing a specific behaviour or issue. Criticism often uses absolute language (like 'always', 'never', 'every time', etc.). Here's an example: 'You're always late. You don't seem to care about anyone else's time other than your own.' Point, shoot and fire. Since criticism is an attack, it's no surprise that it makes people defensive and escalates conflict.

You can manage criticism by offering a constructive complaint. This focuses on a specific behaviour and its impact rather than attacking a person's character. Check out the difference. 'Yesterday when you were late, I was frustrated. I'd organized my morning to be ready and I felt like that wasn't considered. Please give me a heads-up next time.' Criticism can be a 'power over' tactic that hurts someone by attacking their character. An alternative 'power with' behaviour is to provide a constructive complaint.

PRINCIPLE 2 – BALANCE YOUR POWER

#2 DEFENSIVENESS

The second amber flag is defensiveness – when we deflect. Defensiveness usually kicks in as a protective response to criticism and involves making excuses and denying responsibility. It acts as a 'power over' behaviour by launching a counterattack. For example: 'Maybe if you were more adventurous, our sex life wouldn't be so boring.' When we're defensive, we often get caught up in thoughts of fairness and position ourselves as the 'innocent' party.[18]

You can manage defensiveness by using the 'power with' behaviour of taking responsibility. For example: 'I understand our sex might feel a bit routine lately. Let's talk about some new things we could try together.' Managing defensiveness doesn't mean taking the blame for everything, but it does mean acknowledging your part in contributing to a situation. Even better? Stop criticizing each other and avoid defensiveness altogether.

#3 CONTEMPT

The third amber flag is contempt. Contempt is when we express disrespect and superiority over someone else. It shows up as disgust, disdain, condescension, disapproval and judgement. Of all the amber flags, this is the nastiest one, because it uses behaviours like sarcasm, mockery and humiliation to cause harm. Contempt often stems from poor communication, unresolved conflict and a build-up of resentment. We've all felt it, and if we're being honest, we've all dished it out. Contempt looks like backhanded compliments, put-downs or cynical remarks, as well as physical behaviours like eye-rolling, sneering or dismissive gestures.

You can manage contempt with 'power to' behaviours like self-reflection and the ability to forgive, as well as 'power with' behaviours like expressing feelings, active listening and taking responsibility. If you're feeling unsure about how to do all of that, we've got you – we'll cover this together in detail in chapter 8.

#4 STONEWALLING

Last but not least of the amber flags is stonewalling. Stonewalling happens when we shut down communication, refuse to engage and withdraw from a situation. Examples include: ignoring, avoiding, sulking, turning away, giving the silent treatment or obsessively distracting ourselves. Sometimes, stonewalling happens when we're emotionally overwhelmed or flooded. Other times, it can be an attempt to punish someone and/or to regain the upper hand. Gentle reminder: passive aggression is still aggression.

Managing stonewalling involves applying 'power to' behaviours that help you self-regulate. For example, agreeing to take a pause so you can let your system reset. You can also manage it by using 'power with' behaviours like letting each other know whether you need support, solutions and/or space, and by scheduling Weekly Retrospectives (see p. 83).

PRINCIPLE 2 – BALANCE YOUR POWER

IT'S OKAY TO BE A WORK-IN-PROGRESS

There you have some amber flags to look out for and Dr Gottman's 'Four Horsemen': criticism, defensiveness, contempt and stonewalling. Hands up – do any of them sound familiar? I'll admit, I used to be a bit of a stonewaller, and Billie had her battles with defensiveness. Even now we sometimes catch ourselves slipping back into these habits, especially when we're feeling stressed or worn-out.

What about you?

Do you spot any of these behaviours in yourself or others?

If you do, that's okay. Remember, they're incredibly common, and we're all works-in-progress. Having these tendencies doesn't make you a 'bad' person, nor does it mean your relationship is doomed. Let's not get ahead of ourselves and go jumping to the worst-case scenario.

The truth is, a lot of us have never been taught how to express ourselves confidently and kindly, or how to communicate effectively. If you're noticing these patterns in yourself or your relationships, take it as a friendly nudge from us to be mindful of when and where they pop up, so they don't keep sneaking in when they're not wanted or helpful. We've already given you some examples of alternative behaviours to help manage them, and we'll also cover how to improve your communication in chapter 8. If you want to go even deeper into the world of power, and explore how and why certain power dynamics come up, we've included some bonus reads at the end of this chapter.

The green flags: How to nurture your 'power to' and 'power with'

As we mentioned earlier, not all power-related behaviours are bad. Power can also be a force for good – it can be supportive, generative and collaborative. These green flags are all about personal empowerment ('power to') and relationship empowerment ('power with'). They're important to keep in mind because sometimes we take the good stuff for granted and forget to celebrate the wins.

There are many ways to nurture and build your 'power to' and 'power with'. Here are some examples of green flags to keep an eye out for and to give you a lovely reminder that you're on the right track. As a heads-up, we'll also cover them in more detail throughout the book, to help give you an idea of how to do them in practice.

HOW TO NURTURE YOUR PERSONAL POWER

- Prioritize your physical, sexual, mental and emotional health and wellbeing
- Build confidence and security in your abilities and your worth

PRINCIPLE 2 — BALANCE YOUR POWER

- Understand and manage your feelings (without judgement)
- Express your needs and set boundaries
- Make your own decisions and take control of your life
- Strengthen your resilience and ability to bounce back from setbacks and challenges
- Set goals, pursue growth and work towards your dreams for the future
- Build meaningful relationships and join supportive communities
- Do things that bring you joy, and discover what turns you on in sex and in general

HOW TO NURTURE YOUR SHARED POWER

- Value and respect each other's opinions, feelings and boundaries
- Communicate considerately through open and honest dialogue
- Empathize and seek to understand where the other person is coming from
- Share decision-making and have an equal say in what happens
- Build and maintain trust by demonstrating reliability and taking responsibility
- Address disagreements and resolve conflicts constructively and with care

- Recognize power dynamics and hold each other accountable when it comes to being balanced
- Encourage independence and support one another's growth and development
- Regularly express gratitude, appreciation and admiration for each other
- Work together towards common goals and a shared future

Balancing power in real life

When it comes to handling power in our relationships, there's no one-size-fits-all solution. This is true for all types of relationships, whether they're with intimate partners, friends, family or colleagues. What works for one person might not work for another, and that's just the way it is. Healthy relationships aim for balance and ensure that everyone involved feels heard, respected and safe. If you notice imbalances in your relationships or that one person is always in charge, it might be time to have a conversation or to re-evaluate the relationship. Remember, if the power balance is way off and impacting your health and wellbeing (or the health and wellbeing of the other person), prioritize getting care and seek support.

For Billie, dealing with power dynamics after her sexual assault was far from easy. Quite the opposite in fact. It was messy, complex and invalidating, and it led her to depression. However, by strengthening her

PRINCIPLE 2 — BALANCE YOUR POWER

'power to' and 'power with' and pushing back against the company's 'power over', she not only pulled herself through but came out more self-aware, confident and empowered.

Here's how . . .

About eight months after the incident, Robert announced he was starting a private mentorship programme for female employees. When I heard the news, my mind flashed back to the bar and everything else that came with it. Fear jolted through me – I was scared for the mentees. That fear became the momentum I needed to start dealing with my depression, as well as my driving force of change. For the first time, I acknowledged what had actually happened. It wasn't just a drunken mishap; it was sexual assault. This wasn't my fault; it was Robert's. He did it and he was going to do it again – he was grooming us. I no longer felt self-pity; I felt rage. I also felt a duty of care. I didn't want what had happened to me to happen to anyone else ever again. Eight months after Robert sexually assaulted me, I finally went to HR.

Instead of chatting in the office, I asked Joyce if we could step out for a coffee. We sat down at a table facing the shop window. I couldn't bring myself to look at her. She was concerned and gently invited me to share. Tears poured down my cheeks as I leaned my forehead against the glass and wept. It was one of the hardest conversations I've ever had; all I felt was an overwhelming sense of shame.

When I finished talking, she put her hand on my shoulder, and replied, 'First of all, I'm sorry this has happened.' Patting my back, she paused for a moment. She cleared her throat and continued, 'Sometimes when we come into work, we have to put a mask on at the door. There is a "work us" and a "personal us".

Right now, you need to leave the personal side at home and put your work mask on so you can show up and do your job.' As she continued to speak, she didn't say a single thing about Robert or the assault. I felt like an idiot.

The next day at work, Phillip, the head of my department, pulled me in for a meeting. Very quickly, I learned Joyce had shared the details of my assault with the wider team. She'd also done so without my consent.

'We've heard what's happened and we'd like to offer you a role in the New York office. There are a few more women there and we think it would be a good environment for you to continue your career.'

'Okay . . . and what about Robert? What's going to happen with him?'

'Look, the thing is, Robert's a really big earner for us. And, well, this is a bit of a "he says, she says" situation.'

There wasn't much more to say after that.

Later that week, I went back to HR. I told Joyce that I didn't feel like this was a realistic solution – it's not like they could move all of us to New York. I'd come forward not for myself but for the women Robert was recruiting for mentoring. She dismissed my concerns and denied responsibility on the company's part. Angry and frustrated, I used the only card I thought I had left.

'If you're not going to do anything about this then I'm going to go public,' I said.

The change in the atmosphere was immediate.

'If you do that, we will make sure that no one will ever hire you again. Your career will be destroyed, as will any of your opportunities for future employment. We will defend Robert and completely refute that any of this ever happened. Your call.'

And that was it.

PRINCIPLE 2 – BALANCE YOUR POWER

It was clear that the structures that were supposed to be there to protect me had failed – and would likely fail again. In my feelings of helplessness and anger, I realized I needed to somehow find and take back my own power. And yet, despite knowing that nothing about this company was serving me, I didn't have the confidence to leave it yet – I lacked 'power to'.

I was still inexperienced and junior. I was also afraid of the power they had over me, and that if I mis-stepped they would sabotage my future employment opportunities and my career.

Not long after, I saw an advert for a career-change programme called Escape the City. This language resonated perfectly. After attending their Welcome Day, I approached Claire, one of the programme coaches. Without going into the details, I told her about what had happened with Robert and how much I was struggling at work. She looked me in the face, took my hand and told me, 'This may not be the right thing for you, you might need therapy. But if you want to do it, we'll help you, and we'll be with you every step of the way.'

It was the first time that another person had acknowledged what I was feeling and recognized my assault for what it was. I felt validated, I felt seen, and I felt a tiny flickering flame of hope.

Over the next three months, I embarked on my own journey of self-discovery while building an incredible community and getting the support I needed. Through structured exercises, meaningful friendships and counselling, I began to rebuild my inner power and sense of self. Slowly, I started to open up about my experience and to learn how to trust others again.

I also set aside time to explore my beliefs, my strengths and weaknesses, and what gave me energy and brought me joy. A big part of reclaiming my power was figuring out how to be comfortable in my body again, and how to find a way back to my sexual self. That's because, after my sexual assault, I was afraid of my own sexuality. Something that had once brought me power now felt disempowering.

I blamed my sexuality for what had happened. That it had somehow invited it. So to reconnect with my body again, I started going to dance classes. Surrounded by other women, dance empowered me to tap back into my playful side in an environment that was safe and supportive. As I became more comfortable with my body again, I moved towards more sexual forms of self-expression. Nothing left me feeling saucier or sexier than twerking or dancing in heels.

Another big part of reclaiming my personal power had to do with the promise I'd made myself to protect the other women I worked with. I went back to HR. This time, I exercised my 'power to' and 'power with' and I laid out exactly what was going to happen. First, they would formally tell the women in the mentoring programme about Robert. Second, I would switch to the learning and development team, where I would set up the mentoring scheme myself and put the necessary guardrails in place. Then, when I was ready, I'd quit – and I would do so on my terms. They agreed.

My sexual assault was the event that changed everything. It set me on an entirely different course, towards not only my own sexual empowerment but the sexual empowerment of thousands of other women. It was one of the worst experiences of my life, but also one of the most profound. Not everything changed right away or was 'fixed' just like that. Unfortunately, that's just not how we're wired. It was, however, the tipping point and the catalyst for my own journey towards sexual empowerment to come.

*

PRINCIPLE 2 — BALANCE YOUR POWER

Power and your ability to influence comes in all sorts of shapes and sizes. From the personal to the professional, power exists within every relationship you have. Whether it's with an intimate partner, a friend or family member, or colleagues, it's important to understand the different types of power and to know what behaviours — good and bad — to watch out for. By getting the support you need and discovering more about who you are, you can strengthen your resilience, your confidence and your inner 'power to'. This can help protect you from abusive 'power over' behaviours and equip you with the community, knowledge and language to help you push back. The more intuitive your 'power to' and 'power with' behaviours become, the better able you'll be to cultivate healthier and more joyful relationships both in and out of the bedroom.

In practice: Here's how to balance power

Tool #1: Identify and balance power styles

Think about how you typically behave in your romantic relationship(s). Without overthinking it, answer the questions below as honestly as you can. When you're done, score each question based on the rubric that follows.* If you have a partner and feel like it, ask them

---

* This quiz is designed for self-reflection and is not a definitive assessment. If you have concerns about power dynamics in your relationship, consider seeking support from a relationship counsellor or therapist.

to complete the questionnaire as well, and set aside some time to share and chat about your answers.

MAPPING POWER DYNAMICS IN YOUR ROMANTIC RELATIONSHIP(S)

1. When it comes to setting boundaries, who usually takes the lead?
   a. I do
   b. My partner does
   c. We both do equally
2. Who is more likely to initiate a conversation about our relationship goals?
   a. I am
   b. My partner is
   c. We both are equally
3. In our relationship, who generally has the final say?
   a. I do
   b. My partner does
   c. We both have equal say
4. When we face a problem, how do we usually solve it?
   a. I take charge
   b. My partner takes charge
   c. We work on it together
5. Who is more likely to compromise their wants or needs in our relationship?
   a. I am
   b. My partner is
   c. We both compromise equally

PRINCIPLE 2 — BALANCE YOUR POWER

6. When planning activities or outings, whose preferences usually take precedence?
   a. Mine
   b. My partner's
   c. We both consider each other's preferences equally
7. How often do I express my sexual desires and needs openly?
   a. Always
   b. Sometimes
   c. Rarely
8. In discussions about our future, who usually leads the conversation?
   a. I do
   b. My partner does
   c. We both contribute equally
9. Who is more likely to give in during a disagreement to keep the peace?
   a. I am
   b. My partner is
   c. We both are equally
10. How often do we make decisions about our relationship together?
    a. Always
    b. Sometimes
    c. Rarely
11. When it comes to household chores, how is the responsibility divided?
    a. I do most of them
    b. My partner does most of them
    c. We share responsibilities equally

12. Who usually initiates conversations about difficult topics or issues?
    a. I do
    b. My partner does
    c. We both do equally
13. In our relationship, who is more likely to assert their opinion?
    a. I am
    b. My partner is
    c. We both assert our opinions equally
14. How do we handle conflicts or arguments?
    a. I usually back down
    b. My partner usually backs down
    c. We work through them together
15. When making plans for the future, whose vision tends to be prioritized?
    a. Mine
    b. My partner's
    c. We both prioritize each other's visions equally

For each question, assign the following points:

- A = 1 point
- B = 2 points
- C = 3 points

Total score:

- **15–23 points:** Your relationship may have an imbalanced power dynamic, with one of you

PRINCIPLE 2 — BALANCE YOUR POWER

holding more sway. Time to check in and work on levelling the playing field.
- **24–33 points:** Your relationship has a mix of power dynamics. Some parts are nice and balanced, while others could use a tune-up. Focus on cultivating your 'power with'.
- **34–45 points:** Your relationship power dynamics are looking pretty balanced, with both of you having an equal say. Keep it up!

BALANCE AND STRENGTHEN POWER WITH THESE 'HOW TO' CHEAT SHEETS

How to create a more balanced power dynamic and manage 'power over':

- **Swap criticism for complaints:** Ditch the character attacks and instead address a specific behaviour or issue. Even better? Give kudos for what your partner does right.
- **Take responsibility, don't defend:** Rather than launching an attack, reflect on how you've contributed to the situation and identify opportunities to do things differently.
- **Don't let the kitchen sink overflow:** Instead of letting issues (aka 'the dishes') pile up and contempt to build, talk about and work through your frustrations as they arise.
- **Take turns at the helm:** Mix it up when making decisions. Start small – like what's for

dinner – and work up to sharing the load when it comes to bigger decisions.
- **Support solo time:** Encourage each other to explore individual passions and hobbies outside of the relationship so you can strengthen your 'power to'.

How to strengthen your 'power to':

- **Carve out me-time:** Block out some weekly slots for things that refill your cup and give you energy.
- **Practise assertiveness:** Use 'I' statements to express your needs and feelings confidently and kindly. It's about being clear, not confrontational.
- **High-five yourself:** Keep a tally of your successes (big and small) and celebrate your wins so that you get better at ditching negative self-talk and disqualifying the good stuff.
- **Develop coping strategies:** Identify healthy tactics that help you chill out so that you can better manage stress and regulate your emotions.
- **Map out your journey:** Set goals that are specific, measurable, achievable, relevant and time-bound, to build your momentum and create a sense of purpose.

PRINCIPLE 2 — BALANCE YOUR POWER

How to strengthen 'power with':

- **Schedule heart-to-hearts:** Set aside time to touch base about your relationship, talk about how you've been feeling and tackle any issues. It's about keeping the lines open.
- **Practise gratitude rituals:** Kick off or wrap up your day by sharing something you appreciate about each other — celebrate the good.
- **Be each other's fan club:** Actively support and encourage each other's dreams, whether that means showing up to events or offering feedback.
- **Build trust through teamwork:** Have fun doing activities that need you to rely on each other and be in sync, like cooking, rock climbing or a board game.
- **Dream up your future together:** Whether it's a Pinterest list, a vision board or bullet points, jot down shared goals and aspirations for what's ahead.

Tool #2: Do a weekly retrospective

The weekly retrospective is like a little time machine that lets you zoom back to the past week so you can reflect on it and discuss it. You can either do this solo ('power to') or with a partner/group ('power with'). It's all about understanding what went well, what went not-so-well, and what you can improve on going forward. This is a great tool for improving and practising communication in a low-risk way. And yes, you might recognize these questions from your own end-of-chapter check-ins – sneakily, we've already been helping you build this practice without you even knowing it!

Here are your step-by-step instructions:

Every 1–2 weeks, set aside 30–45 minutes to check in with your partner. During this time, you'll each take ten minutes to answer the following:

1. What went well this week in our relationship?
2. What went not-so-well this week in our relationship?
3. What is one thing I/we can do to make next week as good or even better?

While one person shares, the other person listens. As a listener, try to channel your inner detective – be curious, don't interrupt, and keep your judgement to a minimum. Make sure to genuinely thank the other person for sharing when they're done. Once you've both had your say, use the remaining time to chat about what popped up and make some plans for moving forward together.

Some tips:

- Introduce the idea of the retrospective ahead of time. You can frame it like this: 'I've been reading a book about relationships and it talks about doing a weekly check-in. Would you be up for trying it together?'

- If you or your partner feel like it's 'too scripted' or 'not spontaneous' enough, give it a shot anyway. Let's face it, arguments are often unscripted and spontaneous, and they don't always end well.
- Struggling to put your feelings into words on the spot? Jot down your thoughts beforehand.
- Don't discuss your sex and relationship life in bed. Instead, choose somewhere neutral like the living room or when you're out for a stroll.
- Timing is everything. Stay clear of retrospectives when feeling drained, hungry, stressed or rushed.
- Embrace it! This is a chance to get to know a new side of each other, enjoy some quality time together and invest in the growth and future happiness of your relationship.

Tool #3: Complete a joy audit

Last but not least, here's a tool that can help you build your inner 'power to', especially if you've been feeling down or disconnected. Meet the joy audit! It's like a treasure hunt for your energy boosters, so you can discover what matters to you – and turns you on – in life. Picture it as an opportunity to figure out where to spend your time (and where not to) so you can nurture and protect your personal power.

PART I: MAKE YOUR DRAINS VS GAINS LIST

Here are your step-by-step instructions:

1. **Get ready:** Grab a pen and paper or something to write with, and find a cosy spot where you can work without distractions.
2. **Make your columns:** Draw three columns. Label them 'Drain', 'Gain' and 'Neutral'. Alternatively, you can download a template at www.turnyourselfon.co.
3. **Fill them up:**
    a. *Drain column*: Jot down anything that's been sucking your energy dry. Instead of writing 'Work', get specific – like, 'Meetings over thirty minutes'.
    b. *Gain column*: List what's been giving you energy. Rather than 'Date night', be specific. Something like 'Deep chats with [name] during dinner, followed by a movie'.
    c. *Neutral column*: Anything that's been 'meh'? Pop it in here.
4. **Spot the patterns:** Look at your columns. Notice any trends? Maybe certain people or activities are always in the 'Drain' or 'Gain' column.
5. **Plan for change:**
    a. Pick one or two energy-zappers you can cut back on or ditch.

PRINCIPLE 2 — BALANCE YOUR POWER

    b. Choose one or two energy boosters you want to do more often.
    c. From the 'Neutral' bunch, decide if there's something you can improve or let go of to free up more energy.
6. **Make it happen:** Set clear goals for each change you're planning. Write down exactly what you're going to do and when.

PART II: (RE)DISCOVER JOY

Now for the fun part! Pick 3–5 activities that are purely about pleasure and joy. These can be from your 'Gain' column, or any other activity that you've been itching to try. The golden rule? These are not chores or must-dos – they're your want-to-dos. Commit to doing them over the next month.

Look back to look forward

> Take 1–2 minutes to reflect and answer the following questions:
>
> 1. How am I balancing power well?
> 2. How am I not balancing power well?
> 3. What's one action I'm going to start, stop or continue NOW to have a better balance of power in my life?

If you'd like to dive deeper, we've hooked you up with some great resources and downloadable templates at www.turnyourselfon.co.

Cement your learnings

- Power is having influence, and it's a part of every relationship you have.
- When we talk about power in relationships, there are three main types:
  - **'Power over'**: This is when one person has power over another.
  - **'Power to'**: This is your inner personal power, the strength you hold within yourself.
  - **'Power with'**: This is the power you share with someone else or a group.
- Keep an eye out for red flag behaviours that show an abuse of power. These can be physical, sexual, psychological or emotional, stalking, digital and financial. Just because someone might not be aware of these abusive behaviours, it doesn't make them less real.
- Gaslighting is a form of emotional and psychological abuse. It makes the victim doubt their feelings, instincts and sanity. Common gaslighting tactics include withholding, countering, diverting, minimizing, denying, projecting and twisting.

PRINCIPLE 2 — BALANCE YOUR POWER

- Watch out for amber flag behaviours like criticism, defensiveness, contempt and stonewalling. Managing these is key to keeping your relationship stable, long-lasting and healthy.
- Embrace green flag behaviours to strengthen your 'power to' and 'power with'. You can find examples of these on pages 82 and 83.
- If you recognize abusive behaviours in your relationship(s), check out the books on trauma in chapter 6 (see p. 231) and the resources below for more information:
  - Rape Crisis – https://rapecrisis.org.uk
  - Victim Support – https://victimsupport.org.uk
  - Samaritans – https://samaritans.org
  - National Domestic Violence Hotline – https://thehotline.org
  - Rape, Abuse & Incest, National Network (RAINN) – https://rainn.org

Bonus reads

- Robert Greene, *The 48 Laws of Power*
- Dale Carnegie, *How to Win Friends and Influence People: The Only Book You Need to Lead You to Success*
- John Gottman, PhD, and Nan Silver, *The Seven Principles for Making Marriage Work: A Practical Guide from the Country's Foremost Relationship Expert*

- Deborah Vinall, PsyD, LMFT, *Gaslighting: A Step-by-Step Recovery Guide to Heal from Emotional Abuse and Build Healthy Relationships*
- Julia Serano, *Sexed Up: How Society Sexualizes Us, and How We Can Fight Back*
- Mikki Kendall, *Hood Feminism: Notes from the Women That a Movement Forgot*
- Prisca Dorcas Mojica Rodríguez, *For Brown Girls with Sharp Edges and Tender Hearts: A Love Letter to Women of Color*
- Laura Bates, *Everyday Sexism: The Project That Inspired a Worldwide Movement*

Principle 3 – Build Your Self-Confidence*

By reframing your core beliefs and managing your cognitive distortions

Whether we're talking the talk or walking the walk, confidence shapes how we feel about ourselves and how other people feel about us too. The more we build our confidence, the more empowered we are to do what it is we want. It puts that little extra pep in our step.

But here's the thing: despite projecting it on the outside, most of us don't feel all that confident on the inside, especially when it comes to sex. Back in 2021, we ran a big survey with almost 12,000 folks between the ages of 18 and 65. Guess what? Less than one in three felt confident knowing and asking for what they wanted in bed.

And it's not just the numbers that tell the story; it's the thousands of real conversations Billie and I have had too. Here's what some of the women we've worked with have shared:

---

* And self-esteem and self-efficacy.

- *'I want to feel confident expressing what I want or even just knowing what I want, so I can ask for it in bed and enjoy sex again. It's like I've lost touch with who I am and what turns me on.'*
- *'Rejection in dating has knocked my confidence. I don't know what I'm doing wrong and I'm scared of ending up alone.'*
- *'I wish I felt more confident taking charge in the bedroom. I'm not always sure what to do or say to make my partner happy.'*
- *'I'm not feeling great about my body right now and it's making me feel insecure during sex. It'd be nice to feel more present and confident when I'm naked.'*

It's not only the bedroom where our confidence can falter; it can happen in any aspect of our lives. When we're about to have a difficult conversation at work, for example, or going through changes in a relationship, navigating family dynamics or trying something new for ourselves. We might even find ourselves feeling anxious about the idea of being judged, rejected or seen as a failure by those around us, whether we are close to them or not.

Not only that, alongside all the other gender gaps we face as women, it turns out there's a confidence gap too. Research shows that, compared to men, women generally underestimate their abilities and performance.[1] On average, we feel less ready to go for promotions, less qualified for jobs and less able to negotiate a raise.[2] We also rate our skills more negatively, expect to do worse on tests and are more likely to turn down opportunities.[3]

PRINCIPLE 3 — BUILD YOUR SELF-CONFIDENCE

This gap starts early. Boys and girls have similar levels of confidence until about age twelve. But by fourteen, boys' confidence is 27 per cent higher than girls'.[4]

It's not just about our academic or outward performance either. Girls start feeling negatively towards their bodies early on too. Around the world, 54 per cent of girls aged 10–17 aren't happy with their bodies, and six out of ten think they need to look a certain way to succeed.[5] Confidence also varies with sexual orientation, disabilities and race. For instance, studies in the US found that Asian American teens feel worse about themselves than African American, Hispanic or white teens.[6]

So what's the takeaway? A lot of us are struggling, and for many of us, it's been a long battle. If you're nodding your head – hello! We see you. This chapter is about building self-confidence, but it's also about more than that. It's about recognizing that self-confidence is just one part of the puzzle that is 'you'. You also need self-esteem and self-efficacy. By the end of this chapter, you'll understand how they're different and have the knowledge and the tools to start building all three.

Feeling better about who you are starts with you. That's because, of all the relationships you'll ever have, the most important one is the one you have with yourself. Ready to dive in? Let's go.

Confidence case study

We often lump self-confidence, self-esteem and self-efficacy together like they're all the same thing. They're not. To show you how easy it can be to mix them up, Billie's got an experience to share with you.

Billie's story

When we were discussing which stories to include in this chapter, I felt my heart sink for the younger me as I shared an experience from uni with Anna. It has to do with a crisis of confidence, a fear of the future and a belief that I wasn't good enough. To make sense of where this lack of confidence and belief had come from, we need to go back to my teenage years and where it all began . . .

My mum's Italian and fits the stereotype of being a confident, passionate and physically affectionate woman – from an early age I intuitively took after her. As a teenager, I noticed the gregariousness and tactile behaviour that came so naturally to me seemed to get attention from the boys. When I was voted the 'biggest flirt' in school, I considered it a good thing, and I was proud. I saw my flirtatiousness as a core part of my personality and I equated it with my worth. I knew that if I behaved a certain way, I could get others to want me, and I liked that – it made me feel desired. After all, what teenage girl doesn't want to be fancied?

What I didn't realize was that the more I wrapped my value up in being wanted, the more I started to subconsciously believe that it was others who defined my worthiness, not me.

Fast-forward to uni.

I wasn't enjoying my courses, and while I was doing well in them, they didn't excite me. Rather than exploring what I wanted for my future, I'd done what people had told me I should do. Something about the direction I was headed felt off, but I didn't know

PRINCIPLE 3 — BUILD YOUR SELF-CONFIDENCE

what it was or how to change it. I just knew that my gut was telling me it was wrong.

And yet, at the time, everyone else seemed to be having fun and so sure of themselves — so I pretended I was too and that I was fine. While on the outside I projected confidence, on the inside I deeply doubted my worthiness. I was insecure about myself, about my decisions and about what was going to come next. As I got closer to the end of my studies, I became more uncertain of myself and my future and I drifted further away from the things that made me happy. Instead of facing my fears and working through my self-doubt, I avoided them. It was in this crisis of confidence that I went back to the one thing I knew I was good at: being a flirt and getting men to fancy me.

Now's a good time for an interlude on my upbringing. While I had a happy and privileged childhood, I grew up in a more patriarchal family, especially when it came to gender roles. My dad was the principal earner and my mum stayed at home with me and my sister full-time. It was a similar dynamic in my wider family too. At dinners, all the women would be in the kitchen, cooking and washing up, whereas the men would be sitting in the living room having heated debates. I inherited this belief that it was up to my partner to provide for me and it was my duty as a wife to support him.

And so, as my confidence waned, sex became a performance, something I did for validation and to feel good about myself. I knew what I needed to do to be 'great' in bed. I'd pleasure my partners a certain way, make noises a certain way, fake orgasms a certain way. It's not that I didn't enjoy sex, it's that my pleasure was dependent on their *pleasure. I'd worry about whether they were having a fun time, whether they found me sexy, whether I was doing the things they wanted. The simple truth was that sex was more for them than for me. Sure, in the moment it was exciting, but most importantly, it gave me the validation that I was good at something. Even though I was completely unaware of it, sex became a tool that reassured me I was worthy.*

Until it wasn't.

In my teenage years, I'd never really gone through sexual rejection. Then, during my early twenties came a period where I experienced rejection in several different relationships and ended up liking my partners more than they liked me. Looking back, I now understand I was young and naive and those relationships weren't actually all that well-matched anyway. At the time, however, it shook me, and left me feeling like I wasn't good enough and needed to be 'better' to be liked. Rejection made me feel like there was something wrong with me and like I wasn't desirable or worthy.

My confidence dropped even more and so did my standards. Instead of creating mutually respectful relationships, I would pursue men who treated me poorly. I'd put up with disrespectful behaviour like being cheated on, kept secret or ghosted, and I'd use sex as a tool to try to build closeness and to convince them I was good enough. When these relationships failed, my confidence failed with them. I believed if I couldn't even get men to want me – the one thing I'd always been good at – there was little hope for my future.

Towards the end of uni, I met Michael. Michael was the first of my two most important long-term relationships – the second being Seb, my current partner.

Michael was a few years older than me and already had a 'proper job' in London. There was something about him that was different to my previous relationships. Looking back, I think it was that he knew exactly what he wanted and oozed a self-confidence that was intoxicating and reassuring to younger me.

PRINCIPLE 3 — BUILD YOUR SELF-CONFIDENCE

While I didn't recognize it for what it was at the time, being with him made me feel like it wasn't a big deal if I lacked confidence, because he had enough for the both of us.

Michael had a clear vision and plan for his future and so it was okay that I didn't. I didn't need to figure everything out because he already had. I could just tag along with him. All I needed to do was to be the 'fun, sexy girlfriend' and everything would be okay.

So that's what I did.

I attached myself to this incredible man who was so sure of himself and so sure of everything at a period when I wasn't sure of anything.

Without realizing it, I defaulted to these inherited beliefs about what my role — and my future husband's role — was 'meant' to be. I adopted this narrative that I didn't need to build a future for myself, but instead marry and support someone who could build that future for me.

Michael was that someone — or at least I thought he was.

We dated for six years (with a couple of on-and-off periods that you'll hear about later). We built an amazing relationship and got on really well, but as the years rolled on, something still felt like it was missing. In hindsight, I think that something was me. I adapted so much to his life and his sense of self — his hobbies, his routines, his friendships — that I all but left myself behind. I didn't feel confident holding my own in our relationship because he was so assertive and established in his ways. The few times I did suggest activities for us to do, ones that I liked, he wasn't all that open to doing them if they deviated from his own interests. Because Michael was so sure of himself and what he wanted, it felt like he took up a lot of the space in our relationship. It didn't feel like there was any space left for me.

I remember sitting on his bed and looking around his room.

Nothing about the aesthetic appealed to me – in fact, I felt suffocated by it. And yet, I had no idea what I would change. I didn't know what I'd put on his walls or how I'd decorate it differently. Ben Howard was playing in the background. I remember thinking to myself, 'If I have to listen to this song one more time, I'm going to lose my shit' – but, just like his room, I didn't know what to change the music to because I didn't know what music I actually liked.

While it seemed sudden, it had all been very gradual – I was living Michael's life, not my own. Not because he was making me, but because I was deferring to him. Even though I wasn't confident in the alternative yet, I was beginning to resent the idea of Michael being my primary provider and the decision-maker in our relationship. Sometimes it felt like he was my dad more than my partner.

My lack of confidence meant I'd never taken the time to discover my own sense of self. And so I felt a real sense of sadness and longing in those moments, as well as a sort of . . . jealousy. While I loved Michael, I was also envious of him, of the fact that he knew himself so well and had this unwavering belief in what he wanted from his life.

I didn't have the answers to those questions. I couldn't yet say who I was or what I wanted. I didn't recognize the beliefs I had about sex, relationships and my future, nor did I recognize how they were impacting me. All I knew was that something in our relationship was bothering me and had been for a while – just like I'd felt with my courses in uni, something was off. It was as if I was forcing myself to once again fit into a mould that wasn't me. I'd reached the point where I couldn't avoid it any longer. I was at a crossroads; I had to decide whether I would keep following someone else's path or finally start building the confidence to create my own.

PRINCIPLE 3 — BUILD YOUR SELF-CONFIDENCE

The science: What you need to know about self-confidence

A lot of the time, when people talk about being more self-confident, they're talking about something else. Take Billie's experience, for example. Sure, she was struggling with her self-confidence, but it wasn't just about being more confident, she was also wrestling with her self-esteem and self-efficacy. While self-confidence, self-esteem and self-efficacy might seem like they're cut from the same cloth, they're actually quite different. Getting a grip on these differences is key. Otherwise, you might end up trying to build the wrong thing or trying to build the right thing, but in the wrong way. And so, friends, it's time to explore the science.

Self-confidence: 'I am able to'

For all you etymology fans, this one's for you. The word 'self-confidence' is a mix of 'self', derived from the Old English meaning 'one's own person', and 'confidence', originating from the Latin *confidere*, which combines *con* (with) and *fidere* (to trust). To be self-confident means to trust in your ability to do something (even if you've never done it before).[7] Sort of like 'I've got this' vibes. Take teenage Billie for example – she had her flirting skills down and was confident in her ability to get boys to fancy her.

Self-confidence grows with your skills. The better

you get at something, the more self-confident you feel about your ability to do it. The more self-confident you are, the more you're up for learning new skills. When confidence is high, it's a sweet positive feedback loop. In the bedroom, high self-confidence might look like being the one to initiate or say no to sex, voicing your sexual needs, setting sexual boundaries, and giving and receiving feedback on what you find hot and not.

On the flip side, when self-confidence is low, it's a whole other story, like what Billie went through. The less she believed she could do something, the less self-confident she felt and the less likely she was to give it a shot. The less she did or tried, the less able she was to build those skills, and the cycle started all over again. As Billie had experienced in her earlier relationships, low sexual self-confidence meant not expressing her needs or desires, going along with sex even when she wasn't feeling it or taking sexual risks she wasn't all that comfortable with.[8] For many of us, low sexual confidence can also look like shutting ourselves off from potentially pleasurable experiences, or not trying something new because we're scared we're going to get it wrong. This is also where our self-confidence can be influenced by our self-esteem.

Self-esteem: 'I am worthy'

Dusting off the old Latin again, 'self-esteem' comes from *aestimare*, meaning 'to value or determine the worth' of something. To have self-esteem means you value yourself as a person. It's that inner feeling of

PRINCIPLE 3 – BUILD YOUR SELF-CONFIDENCE

worthiness – not only about what you can do, but about who you are. Your self-esteem is packed full of all those warm fuzzy feelings like self-respect, self-compassion and self-love. When our self-esteem is high, we see ourselves in a positive light and are able to build more balanced and healthier relationships.

But when our self-esteem takes a hit, it can be tough. We might start doubting our worthiness – questioning whether we're good enough, wanted by others or deserving of love. We also doubt whether we are worthy and deserving of pleasure. It's like a big dark cloud of 'not enough' and 'should' thoughts floating around in our heads. Over time, these thoughts can turn into deep-rooted beliefs that make us question whether we're 'normal' or 'broken'.

Here's the kicker: women are not just facing a confidence gap, we're facing a self-esteem gap too. A 2016 study involving over 980,000 people across forty-eight countries found men generally had higher self-esteem than women.[9] Looking back at Billie's story, you can see her lack of self-esteem in action. Our self-esteem can take a hit when we base our worth on how others perceive us rather than how we feel about ourselves.

Self-esteem is different from self-confidence. It's about how you feel about yourself as a person, not just your abilities. That's why flipping through *Cosmo*'s 'Top 5 Positions to Spice Up Your Sex Life' might not do a lot to build your self-esteem. And as we saw with Billie, you can be self-confident in one thing but still struggle with self-esteem. Or you might have high self-esteem but low self-confidence. Both combinations are not only possible, but common.

Self-efficacy: 'I can achieve my dreams'

Last but not least, let's talk about self-efficacy. This is about believing in your ability to hit your goals, create your future and achieve your dreams.[10] It's the conviction that your efforts and actions can get you to where you want to be.[11] Billie, for instance, felt she needed to marry Michael to secure her future, mistakenly thinking it was only self-confidence that she lacked, when it was also self-efficacy (and self-esteem).

Self-efficacy is shaped by our beliefs and past experiences. Billie's inherited belief that as a woman, she needed to rely on a husband to support her – combined with her experiences of rejection by men in her twenties – left her doubting her ability to achieve her goals and create her own future, resulting in low self-efficacy. In reality, Michael wasn't the cause of her lack of self-efficacy, but the result of it.

Having self-efficacy and taking control of your future doesn't mean that you'll never mess up. It means that you trust yourself to learn and course-correct when needed. Whether in or out of the bedroom, high self-efficacy looks like regulating your behaviour – for example, learning how to manage negative self-talk or how to get a grip on your inner critic, as well as getting to the root of unhelpful behaviours like procrastination, perfectionism and avoidance.

It also looks like keeping your motivation up and

PRINCIPLE 3 — BUILD YOUR SELF-CONFIDENCE

finding ways to stay inspired and focused, whether through celebrating small milestones, seeking support from others or creating a weekly or monthly practice of reviewing your long-term goals, be they personal, professional, financial, sexual, etc.

Last but not least, you can build self-efficacy by creating conditions that set you up for success, like minimizing distractions, getting a mentor, role model or coach, and organizing your physical environment in a way that helps you rather than impedes you. Some examples? Not sleeping with your phone by your bed; tidying and creating clutter-free spaces; and developing rituals or cues – like going for a walk, having a shower, writing a list – to signal the start and end of different activities so you can better transition between them.

Your self-confidence, self-esteem and self-efficacy all play a part in shaping your sense of self. While they're different concepts, feeling good about yourself, across all areas of your life, requires nurturing and building all three.

QUICK TIP

Next time you catch yourself thinking about being more confident, ask yourself, 'What do I need this confidence for?'

If your answer is about mastering a skill or feeling more capable of doing something, then yep, it's

> confidence you should be focusing on. But if your answer digs deeper and touches on feelings of worthiness, being wanted, and feeling connected or loved, it's time to work on building your self-esteem. And if it's about believing in your future or your ability to hit your goals and achieve your dreams, take a look at your self-efficacy.

Core beliefs: Just because you think it, doesn't make it true

At the heart of developing your self-confidence, self-esteem and self-efficacy are your core beliefs. These are the assumptions and biases you have about who you are and how the world works – a common one in the bedroom is 'their pleasure comes first'.

Imagine your brain as a supercomputer designed to help you make sense of the world and your place in it. It's constantly processing and organizing information in a way that you can understand. Most of this goes on in your unconscious mind, where all the things you're not aware of reside – feelings, desires, memories, etc. These come together to form stories, or beliefs, about who you are and how you see the world.

Because we're not fully aware of all this unconscious activity, it's tough to separate out our perceptions of the world from how the world actually is. It's easy to mistake our beliefs for facts. A fact is an objective truth,

PRINCIPLE 3 – BUILD YOUR SELF-CONFIDENCE

independent of personal opinion, verifiable through evidence and universally accepted. For example, when a person is aroused, their heart rate increases – that's a fact.

A belief, on the other hand, is an assumption you make about what's 'true' or what 'exists' – like 'masturbation is dirty' or 'sex is only good if it ends in orgasm'. These are beliefs, not facts.

Beliefs are basically strong opinions shaped by past experiences, feelings and knowledge. This is part of the reason they feel so deeply 'true'. They're also influenced by – and often inherited from – family, friends, social and cultural institutions, and the media. For instance, Billie inherited the belief that it was up to her partner to provide for their family and it was her duty as a wife to support them. When our beliefs are challenged, our brain interprets it as a threat not only to our identity, but to everything we know about the world. Needless to say, it can feel pretty jarring.

Cognitive distortions: How your brain accidentally sabotages you

By this point, it's pretty clear your brain plays a major role in how you feel about yourself, both in and out of the bedroom. As we often hear from sex educators and therapists, sex happens between your ears, not between your legs. But as amazing as your brain is, it can sometimes take shortcuts and make mistakes. That's where cognitive distortions come into play.

Cognitive distortions are patterns of irrational, automatic and destructive thoughts – essentially, the brain's 'thinking errors'. They occur when our brains misinterpret something, leading us to view situations or experiences in a negative and 'distorted' way. If left unchecked, these little tricksters can interfere with our relationship with ourselves, with others and with the world in general.

There are fifteen common cognitive distortions. If Billie and I were the betting types, we'd wager that you, like everyone else, have quite a few of them. You might even recognize some in Billie's story.

Now, fifteen is a lot – we don't expect you to memorize all these cognitive distortions or know them by heart. That's not really the point. Instead, we suggest you put a tick next to any that resonate with you in the list below, and bookmark this page for future reference.

15 COMMON COGNITIVE DISTORTIONS OR 'THINKING ERRORS'

- __ **All-or-nothing thinking:** Viewing situations as black or white rather than a continuum. Example: 'Either I'm right or wrong.'
- __ **Overgeneralization:** Making broad conclusions based on a single event. Example: 'I was rejected before so I'm going to be rejected again.'
- __ **Mental filtering:** Focusing on the negative details and ignoring the positive ones. Example: 'Even though I enjoyed having it, the sex was bad because I didn't come.'

PRINCIPLE 3 – BUILD YOUR SELF-CONFIDENCE

- __ **Disqualifying the positives:** Rejecting positive experiences by insisting they 'don't count', and dismissing compliments. Example: 'They're just saying that to be nice.'
- __ **Jumping to conclusions:** Making negative interpretations without actual evidence. This happens in two main ways . . .
  - __ **Mind-reading:** Assuming you know what others are thinking. Example: 'She hasn't replied to my message, she must be upset with me.'
  - __ **Fortune-telling:** Predicting things will turn out badly. Example: 'I can't apply for that – I won't get an interview because I'm not qualified enough.'
- __ **Magnifying (catastrophizing) or minimizing:** Making situations bigger or smaller.
  - __ **Magnifying:** Exaggerating an issue and jumping to the worst-case scenario. Example: 'We don't have sex as much as we used to, our relationship is over.'
  - __ **Minimizing:** Downplaying a situation and making it less relevant. Example: 'I'm fine, it's not a big deal.'
- __ **Emotional reasoning:** Believing that because you feel a certain way, it must be true. Example: 'I feel guilty, so I must be guilty.'
- __ **'Should' statements:** Using 'should', 'ought to' or 'must' as self-imposed rules for yourself and others. Example: 'I should go to the gym' or 'I shouldn't have to ask'.

__ **Labelling and mislabelling:** Assigning global, negative labels to oneself or others. Example: 'I'm not good enough' or 'Masturbation is dirty'.

__ **Personalization:** Believing that you are responsible for things outside of your control or that everything is personal. Example: 'It's up to me to make sure they enjoy themselves.'

__ **Blaming:** Holding others responsible for your own emotional pain. Example: 'I don't enjoy sex because my partner doesn't do it right.'

__ **Fallacy of fairness:** Believing that life should always be fair even when fairness is subjective, unrealistic or not possible. Example: 'I expect my partner to know what I'm thinking without having to explain it. It's not fair that I always have to spell it out.'

__ **Control fallacies:** Believing one has complete control over every event (internal control fallacy) or no control at all (external control fallacy). Example: 'It's entirely up to me to fix it.'

__ **Fallacy of change:** Expecting others to change to suit your needs and desires. Example: 'If they love me, they'll change and everyone will be happy.'

__ **Heaven's-reward fallacy:** Believing that suffering and self-sacrifice will eventually pay off. Example: 'If I sacrifice now, it'll be worth it later.'

PRINCIPLE 3 – BUILD YOUR SELF-CONFIDENCE

So, did we guess right?

Were there a lot of cognitive distortions that resonated with you?

If so, that's great! It's useful information to have. Sure, looking at this list might feel intimidating, overwhelming and even disheartening at first – and that's okay. The good news is that you now know what you need to work on to manage unhelpful thoughts and overthinking, so that you can build your self-confidence and sense of self-worth. The goal isn't to control or eliminate every single thought you have – that's not realistic. Instead, the goal is to be aware of common thought patterns you have and explore how they show up for you. Confidence isn't about being perfect, it's about trusting yourself to try. It's also about accepting what's in your control and starting to let go of all the stuff that's not. Don't worry, to help get you started, we've got some great tools for you at the end of this chapter.

Building self-confidence (and self-esteem and self-efficacy) in real life

We've said it before and we'll say it again: the most important relationship you'll ever have is the one you have with yourself. You don't have to love every inch of yourself all of the time – that's a lot of pressure. But if you do want to feel better about yourself and build your confidence day-to-day, it's essential to get to know your worth, what your skills are and what you're working towards so that you can accept the good, the bad and everything in between.

When Billie and I talked about how she went from lacking self-confidence, self-esteem and self-efficacy to having a more positive sense of self and becoming sexually empowered, here's what she shared:

My relationship with Michael started to fully break down in the immediate aftermath of my sexual assault, a period when my self-confidence hit an all-time low. Here's why . . .

The lingering questions from my university days resurfaced. I wasn't confident in my sexual self or my professional self, and I'd thought my doubts had been silenced by being with Michael. It turned out they were still there, demanding answers.

Who was I in my sexual and romantic relationships, and what was my role? Who was I professionally and how could I provide for myself? What did I want for my future? Was I on a path that was fulfilling and making me happy? What did it mean to be empowered – and was I?

Recognizing how low my confidence had sunk, I adopted a new approach. Instead of seeking validation from others, I focused on building it from within.

This meant seeing myself as a sort of . . . blank slate, and redefining my beliefs and desires on my own terms. I reflected on my different selves – my sexual self, my romantic self, my personal self, my professional self, my future self – and I started pulling them into a 'single self': Billie. This meant prioritizing areas that I'd previously neglected or avoided, especially when it came to sex and relationships, my career and my future.

Starting with sex and relationships, I realized how uneducated

PRINCIPLE 3 — BUILD YOUR SELF-CONFIDENCE

I was about sex and how limited my understanding of sexuality was.

For example, I used to carry a lot of shame around masturbating. I remember when one of my friends offered to let me borrow her vibrator, I was shocked. First that this woman actually owned a sex toy, and second that she was so casual in suggesting I borrow it to have a wank. I hadn't understood the point of solo sex, as sex had always been about others' pleasure, not mine.

But as I worked on cultivating my sexual self-confidence and self-esteem, my perspective shifted. It wasn't through my partners that I started to discover myself, but through my own sexual exploration.

Masturbation became a safe way for me to connect with my sexuality and to build my sexual self-confidence by practising how to give myself pleasure and to do so for no one other than me. I also realized that if I didn't know how to touch my own body, I'd struggle to ask for how I wanted it to be touched by others. I learned I didn't need external validation from a sexual partner to feel worthy of respect, love and pleasure — that power already existed within myself.

*While I was cultivating my sexual self-confidence and self-esteem, I was also working to build those same qualities in my professional life. I mentioned in an earlier chapter that I joined a career-change programme called Escape the City. A big part of the programme was about reflecting on our past selves to gain insight into our future selves. In doing so, two beliefs stood out for me: 'My **value** comes from making myself desirable and being good in bed' and 'I don't need to build a **future** for myself, but to marry and support someone who can build that future for me'.*

'Value' and 'future'. These words kept cropping up everywhere. When they did, they filled me with uncertainty and apprehension.

Lucky for me, one of the first exercises we did was to visualize the future we wanted and compare it to our current reality. The disconnect was real. One, because where I was, was pretty shit. And two, while I couldn't yet articulate the future I wanted, I could feel that the direction I was headed wasn't it. So, I leaned into the uncertainty and the apprehension and I set out to explore it. This is where building my self-efficacy came in and why Michael and I finally called it quits.

The more I began to discover myself and my potential through guided exercises as part of the programme, the more I realized the future that I'd thought I'd wanted with Michael wasn't the future I wanted at all. I remember my grandfather telling me to settle down with Michael because 'he's a good guy and a solid bet'. It was the word 'bet' that stood out to me. Like I was taking a gamble on my life rather than taking command of it or asserting my agency.

The more I got to know myself – both sexually and professionally – and the more I built my sense of self, the more I realized it was time for Michael and me to end things once and for all. It wasn't that he was a bad person or that there was anything wrong with our relationship – he was an amazing partner and we got along wonderfully. It was that I was no longer the person I was when we'd gotten together six years ago, and our visions of the future were no longer aligned. Staying together would have meant abandoning my newfound sense of self and the version of me I was becoming.

Building my self-confidence, self-esteem and self-efficacy not only empowered me to end things with Michael, but also to resign from work. For the first time in my adult life, I was starting to believe that I was capable of deciding my own path, creating my own future and achieving my own successes. It was a major tipping point.

PRINCIPLE 3 — BUILD YOUR SELF-CONFIDENCE

The growth that followed was life-changing. I launched myself into it all. I trained as a qualified health coach, I co-founded Ferly, and I gave my first TEDx talk. I promise you, it was a real test of confidence to get on stage and talk to hundreds of strangers (and my dad) about sex.

Through educating myself and educating others, I have created my own definition of sexual empowerment — one that feels authentic to me. Sex is no longer a performance, but a practice. One that gives me the opportunity to both explore and express myself and to do so either on my own or together with another person, as equals.

For me, I can feel the manifestation of my confidence in my ability to have honest and open conversations about sex. I still remember Dad spitting his coffee all over the table when I asked Mum how often she masturbated. By talking about sex, going to events and learning about sexuality, I've developed the skills to be in command of my full self in different environments. More than that, I've learned how to play with my sexuality in a way that feels good and brings me joy.

If there is one thing I know with certainty, it's that our sexualities are a living breathing part of who we are. Sex is a powerful tool for self-discovery. I see it as a window into who I am, how I'm feeling and what I need, not only in my relationships but across all areas of my life. I believe that if we want to be truly empowered, we need to be sexually empowered too. The key to this is building our self-esteem, self-efficacy and self-confidence.

Billie's experiences show that by developing all three aspects of ourselves, we can believe in our ability to succeed, feel worthy and see ourselves as capable of shaping our future. This comes from understanding the differences between self-confidence, self-esteem and self-efficacy, so you can prioritize the areas of your life that might need a little more attention, as well as identifying and reframing your limiting beliefs and managing your cognitive distortions. Sex can and should be a tool for self-discovery and a window into who you are. Learning how to cultivate and nurture your confident sexual self can help you see through that window and lead to a healthier, more confident and more pleasurable life overall.

In practice: Here's how to build self-confidence (and self-esteem and self-efficacy)

Tool #1: Reframe your beliefs

Reframing your core beliefs is all about recognizing, challenging and changing beliefs that are often negative and limiting. It's like taking control back from your inner critic. This is an excellent tool for boosting your self-esteem.

Here are your step-by-step instructions:

1. **Identify a core belief you want to change:** Start by making a list of up to five beliefs that negatively impact your life. These might be about sex but they might not. Here are some examples from our community:

PRINCIPLE 3 — BUILD YOUR SELF-CONFIDENCE

- *'I'm not [X] enough.'*
- *'It takes too long for me to come.'*
- *'Masturbation isn't for me.'*
- *'If I don't look a certain way, people won't find me attractive.'*
- *'I don't know how to be alone.'*
- *'It's selfish to do things for myself.'*

2. **Trace the origin:** Start with one of your beliefs and reflect on when and where it comes from. This helps to demystify its power.
   - For example, one of the origins of Billie's belief that 'I need to marry well to be financially supported' came from gender roles and communication patterns she had observed in her family and her own upbringing.
3. **Evaluate the belief:** Examine the evidence supporting and contradicting this belief. Remember that just because you believe it, doesn't make it true. Ask yourself, 'Is this belief always true?' and 'What evidence do I have that shows otherwise?'
4. **Consider the impact:** Reflect on how this belief has affected your life. How would your life be different otherwise? Think about decisions you've made (and not made) and how the belief has influenced your thoughts, feelings and behaviours.
5. **Challenge the belief:** Now for the fun part. Play devil's advocate. Your role is to challenge the 'truth' of this core belief with counter-evidence.

For each piece of evidence you can think of that supports your belief, find an instance or fact that contradicts it. Write these down.
6. **Develop an alternative belief:** Here's where you get to flip the script. Based on your reflection and the evidence against your core belief, come up with an alternative one that's more balanced, flexible and empowering.
    - Example: 'My value is more than being successful with men. I'm capable of creating my own future and will find success in many ways.'
7. **Gather evidence for your new belief:** Use your bias in a good way. Actively look and filter for evidence that supports your new, positive belief. Evidence might be feedback from others, situations you've witnessed, advice you'd give someone, stories from friends, etc.
8. **Practise your new belief:** This step is important. It's all about creating new patterns and associations in your brain. Integrate your new belief into your daily life. Use affirmations, journaling or visualization to reinforce it and help it stick. Notice situations that support your new belief, as well as situations that challenge it. Keep track of these, and reflect on them as you go.

Tool #2: Challenge your cognitive distortions

A thought diary is a handy tool for identifying, tracking and challenging your cognitive distortions. It's also great

PRINCIPLE 3 – BUILD YOUR SELF-CONFIDENCE

for self-soothing and regulating when you're feeling stuck in your head, and it can help you build both self-esteem and self-confidence. It only takes a minute and you can do it anywhere – on your phone, in a notebook, even in your head. You'll find downloadable templates at www.turnyourselfon.co.

Here is a template for you to follow with prompts and examples of answers:

The situation or trigger was . . .	Being rejected
My immediate feelings, thoughts and behaviours are . . .	Feelings: *Worthlessness, fear, sadness, jealousy* Thoughts: *I'm not even capable of doing this one thing right; I'm not good enough; I need to make myself more desirable; If I can't keep a man how am I going to have a secure future* Behaviours: *Propositioning myself, performative sex, faking orgasms, seeking validation*
The types of distortions I'm having are . . .	*All-or-nothing thinking, catastrophizing, mislabelling, personalization*

Evidence for my thought(s) . . .	*I was cheated on*
Evidence against my thought(s) . . .	*There's plenty of reasons why people decide relationships aren't working and I don't actually know why they did what they did;* *I have an otherwise successful track record with dating;* *I'm good at a lot of things other than sex, e.g. sport, public speaking, managing people;* *Lots of women choose to stay at home and lots of women choose to work, neither choice is right or wrong, they're just different and any future is possible*
A more balanced thought might be . . .	*I am both capable and worthy as a person and there are other ways to feel secure in myself and my future beyond getting men to fancy me*

Tool #3: Manifest your future

This tool is all about boosting your self-efficacy by focusing on your sense of purpose. It encourages you

PRINCIPLE 3 — BUILD YOUR SELF-CONFIDENCE

to get clear about the activities you enjoy, your values and strengths, as well as the impacts you want to make. Feel free to use it to explore your sexual self, relationship self, career self, personal self or any other aspect of yourself you'd like to know better. You'll want to set aside 15–30 minutes (or more) to do this exercise. You'll also need somewhere to make notes that you can easily refer back to in the future.

Here are your step-by-step instructions:

1. **Reflect on pleasurable activities:** Write down things you enjoy doing, both now and in the past. For example: lying in the sun, sipping a cup of tea or coffee, being in nature, being active, doing crafts, reading a book, listening to music, taking a bath, spending time with friends, having a long make-out or cuddling on the couch.
2. **Identify 5–10 core values:** Write down 5–10 values that are important to you. Examples include: intimacy, equality, curiosity, playfulness, autonomy, empathy, growth, security.
3. **Explore your strengths:** Using verbs, make a list of your skills and talents whether in the bedroom or beyond. Think about what you're good at and what others admire in you. Bedroom examples: giving a massage, initiating sex, building anticipation, being attentive. Other examples: problem-solving, empathizing, collaborating, organizing, creating, adapting, communicating.

4. **Visualize your ideal relationship or world:** Imagine your ideal relationship or world where you're happy and fulfilled. Get started by describing who you're with, what you're doing and how you measure success, and end with 1–2 lines describing how you feel.
5. **Create a purpose statement:** Write a statement that summarizes your purpose in life or in a relationship. Start with phrases like 'I am here to . . .' and keep it clear and concise.
6. **Set some goals:** Based on your reflections, set 1–3 small, attainable goals for the next 1–3 months. Make sure they're specific, measurable, achievable, relevant and time-bound (aka SMART).
7. **Reflect and adjust regularly:** Regularly check in to see if your life and/or relationship aligns with your purpose statement and goals. Adapt it if you need to over time.

Look back to look forward

Take 1–2 minutes to reflect and answer the following questions:

1. How am I building my sense of self-confidence, self-esteem and self-efficacy?
2. How am I not building my sense of self-confidence, self-esteem and self-efficacy?

PRINCIPLE 3 — BUILD YOUR SELF-CONFIDENCE

> 3. What's one action I'm going to start, stop or continue NOW to have more self-confidence, self-esteem and self-efficacy in my life?
>
> If you'd like to dive deeper, we've hooked you up with some great resources and downloadable templates at www.turnyourselfon.co.

Cement your learnings

- **Self-confidence:** Trusting in your ability to succeed in doing something, even if you haven't done it before.
- **Self-esteem:** Valuing yourself and deeming yourself worthy as a person.
- **Self-efficacy:** Believing that you are capable of hitting your goals, creating your future and achieving your dreams.
- **Beliefs:** The assumptions you make and the thoughts you have that something is 'true' or 'exists'. They are not the same as facts. A fact is an objective truth that exists independent of personal opinion, and is verifiable through evidence and universally accepted. A belief is a strong opinion or assumption. Just because you believe something, that doesn't make it true.
- **Limiting beliefs:** Assumptions or thoughts that are disempowering and can negatively impact your self-confidence, self-esteem and self-efficacy.

- **Cognitive distortions:** Sometimes your brain takes shortcuts, leading to automatic, irrational and destructive thinking patterns. These are a distorted and often negative view of reality and can also impact your self-confidence, self-esteem and self-efficacy. There are fifteen common ones (see p. 106).

Bonus reads

- Gloria Steinem, *Revolution from Within: A Book of Self-Esteem*
- Peggy Orenstein, *Girls and Sex: Navigating the Complicated New Landscape*
- Brené Brown, PhD, LMSW, *I Thought It Was Just Me (But It Isn't): Making the Journey from 'What Will People Think?' to 'I Am Enough'*
- Katty Kay and Claire Shipman, *The Confidence Code: The Science and Art of Self-Assurance – What Women Should Know*
- Sonya Renee Taylor, *The Body Is Not an Apology: The Power of Radical Self-Love*
- Lindsay Kite, PhD, and Lexie Kite, PhD, *More Than a Body: Your Body Is an Instrument, Not an Ornament*
- Sally Winston, PsyD, and Martin Seif, PhD, *Overcoming Unwanted Intrusive Thoughts: A CBT-Based Guide to Getting Over Frightening, Obsessive or Disturbing Thoughts*

Principle 4 – Cultivate Your Intimacy

By identifying your attachment style and expressing your intimate needs

Defining intimacy can be like defining love. Because it's shaped by our background, attachment style and intimate needs, it's different for everyone. Yet, just like love, we expect everyone to know exactly what we mean when we talk about it. When we say we want more intimacy, what are we really after? Is it about having sex more often, spending quality time together, hearing words of affirmation? At its heart, intimacy is about more than sex. It's about creating a deep and meaningful connection, which lays the foundation for sex (and more).[1] We cultivate it by sharing experiences, feelings, conversations, touch – each different but important in its own way. Intimacy doesn't pop up out of nowhere; it's built through connection, respect and trust. It's not something that exists, it's something you do.

More than money issues or infidelity, a lack of intimacy is one of the most frequent causes for why couples seek therapy.[2] With nearly half of marriages ending in divorce, it's clear that many of us are struggling to meet our intimate needs.[3] Plenty of research studies also show that a lack of intimacy doesn't just impact your relationship satisfaction, but your sexual satisfaction and desire too.[4] For example, how interested you are in sex relates to how connected and responsive you perceive your partner to be. If you have a partner who understands and respects your intimate needs, you are more likely to want to have sex with them. On the flip side, if your partner isn't meeting your intimate needs, you might not feel so inclined to have it. In publications like the *Journal of Sex Research* and the *Journal of Sex and Marital Therapy*, there are some substantial studies to back this up, showing that more intimacy leads to increases in sexual desire, sexual activity and overall relationship satisfaction.[5]

In this chapter, we'll explore what intimate needs are, where they come from and how you can feel good about figuring out and sharing your own. By the time we're done, you'll see that intimacy isn't a by-product of your relationship, but a real biological need. You'll also learn about different attachment styles and how intimate needs vary for each. You'll then get the chance to identify your own attachment style, and explore how you define intimacy and what it means to you. Intimacy matters because, without it, our connections fall apart. But fear not – by the end of this chapter you'll know what you need to know about intimacy to make sure your relationships stay as connected as the world's best Wi-Fi.

PRINCIPLE 4 — CULTIVATE YOUR INTIMACY

Intimacy case study

Now for some hard truths. By definition, it's not intimacy if only one person is doing the work — you can't build a meaningful connection if there's no one to connect to. Since we all have our own idea of what intimacy feels like, what works for you might not be the same for someone else. That's why it's important to know and share your own intimate needs, while also being open to the needs of others.

To give you an idea of how things can go sideways when our expectations of intimacy don't align, I want to share a story from my own dating life — one that kept happening over and over again.

Anna's story

Before I knew what attachment styles were and how they affect our intimate needs (more on this later), I spent years swinging between two extremes in my relationships. Neither was good for anyone involved, and given that I was so involved in them, I couldn't see how contradictory they were. For a long time, I thought something was wrong with me because I couldn't seem to settle for the same 'normal' things as everyone else. Then one night, it all caught up with me . . .

It was dark, sometime after midnight. I was biking home and the streets were quiet except for the rain and the occasional bus that swooshed by. In front of me, the streetlamps cast these eerie yellow reflections across the wet road, creating a scene straight from a Victorian Gothic. I was coming back from Calum's place.

We'd met for a drink at the pub and headed to his. Every time was the same. We'd hover in his kitchen and make small talk, argue about how to make a proper cup of tea, and he'd move to unzip my jeans. I'd lean back against the countertop, and next to a half-full dish rack and a roll of kitchen towel, he'd finger me for a minute or two. Then, he'd throw me over his shoulder, carry me to his room and we'd fuck.

To be honest, I don't think he knew how to do much else. At first, I was kind of into it. It matched up with what I was taught 'hot sex' was supposed to be. And truth be told, it was actually pretty hot. For the first few times at least. Then, all the scripted-ness of bang-bang-banging got boring. It started to feel like I was a prop for him to re-enact something from PornHub.

He also had so many unspoken rules. He only kissed me once – after our first date. Since then, nothing. I likened him to a millennial hipster version of Julia Roberts in Pretty Woman. 'No kissing, it's too personal.' In addition to not kissing, he never touched my hands. As if touching them was too close to holding them and holding them was too close to real intimacy. Being inside of me though – apparently that wasn't. Oral was also off the table. Well, him receiving it was fine. I'd asked him about that once and he'd told me he only went down on girlfriends. I guess our eleven months of sleeping together didn't qualify.

After sex, Calum would immediately flop onto his back, naked except for a pair of white socks, and spread out like a starfish. Instead of cuddling, he'd check his phone in silence. He wasn't big on me hanging around after so I'd get up and dress while he replied to his messages. He'd then hop in the shower and yell something inaudible about getting home safe as I let myself out. In almost a year, he'd never asked me to stay over.

I wasn't stupid, I knew what this was and I also knew it

PRINCIPLE 4 — CULTIVATE YOUR INTIMACY

would never work. I also didn't even want it to — he was too distant and too disinterested, and we had nothing in common. It was the fact that he'd never asked me to stay though — that was what bothered me. It felt like he was unaware that I was not a hook-up, but a person. One who had feelings and who might want to spend the night, especially knowing I had to cycle home in the pissing rain. And so, every time we hooked up, I'd leave feeling used, discarded and humiliated. More than that, I'd feel ashamed — not of Calum but of myself, for doing it again.

In the days after, my shame would turn to insecurity. Like I'd knowingly given him permission to disrespect me, and in doing so, I'd knowingly disrespected myself. I'd check my phone to see if he'd messaged me. I'd open Instagram to see when he'd last been online. I'd post something about where I was hanging out, hoping he'd swing by or reach out. He never did.

In all the time we were 'together', I never brought up my feelings or what I wanted sexually. I knew his type and I didn't want to scare him off. I didn't want to be in a relationship with him but something about being rejected and replaced by one of the other women he was seeing set me off.

So I soothed my insecurities and sought intimacy elsewhere. I'd reach out to the other men I had on the go, like Marcus. Marcus was the opposite of Calum. When I was feeling insecure and needed to feel worshipped and adored, Marcus was my man. He didn't hook up, he made love. Marcus was romantic. He'd make me dinner, plan amazing dates and leave poems tied to my bike. When it came to sex, Marcus would spend an entire evening kissing me, touching me, going down on me, never expecting anything in return. His sole focus was my pleasure. As our bodies eventually entwined, he'd wrap his fingers in mine, look me in my eyes and kiss me as he came. In the afterglow, we'd lie together, my head resting on his chest and him tracing my shoulder while he whispered all the ways he found me sexy.

While he was kind and generous and attentive, eventually his intensity made me feel claustrophobic and trapped. I'd be overwhelmed by a visceral feeling of 'ick' and the need to escape. I'd make an excuse about how I had to go, which left him silent and sulking. With Marcus, I'd leave feeling frustrated, suffocated and overwhelmed. I knew this relationship wasn't going anywhere either – his affection was too pushy, too demanding, too much.

In the days after Marcus and I made love, I needed space. I needed to feel like I had freedom, independence and autonomy. I needed to feel like I was a person, not something for him to consume. He'd WhatsApp me, and if I didn't reply, he'd call, and if I didn't answer, he'd message me on Facebook or Instagram. I'd be deeply uncomfortable by how persistent he was, which made me feel like I needed even more space. Instead of seeing him as romantic, I saw him as intense. Instead of feeling adored, I felt smothered. I knew I was being unfair to him, and I felt guilty and like a total asshole. Still, I dreaded having to see him because I knew he'd want to have yet another 'talk' about our 'situation'. We'd already had several, each of which left me feeling more drained, more distant and more turned off than the last.

Plus, while I was distancing myself from Marcus, Calum had messaged me and said he wanted to grab a drink. Obviously, I said sure.

And so, here I was, cycling home after yet another unsatisfying hook-up through streets that felt as empty as I was. I wasn't happy in my sex or dating life; I hadn't been for a long time. I kept using sex as a way to bring me closer to whatever it was I was looking for. Anything felt better than the nothingness I felt otherwise. I was never satisfied though – what came with it was either way too little *or way too much. I knew things weren't working. If I were being honest with myself, I think somewhere deep inside, I knew that it was **because** they weren't working that I kept these relationships alive. It felt safer that way, like having an emergency exit.*

It was on that ride home, weaving through London's empty streets at night, that I realized I had no idea what real intimacy was. I'd thought it was the closeness that happened during sex, but that was so fleeting and shallow. I was wrong; I had to be. Surely intimacy was something more. But I didn't know, because I'd never taken the time to know my intimate self. Despite riding home through a city packed with more than eight million people, I'd never felt so alone.

The science: What you need to know about intimacy

Now, you might have heard a bit about attachment styles – they're all the rage as of late. However, Billie and I want to make sure you also know what an attachment style actually is. That's because we're all about understanding the 'why' behind science, not just the 'what'. Sound good? Let's get into it.

The way we experience intimacy now has a lot to do with our childhood. Growing up, the quality of relationship you had with your caregiver(s) will have shaped how you cope and what you need in your close relationships as an adult. This is what we call an attachment style.

There are four main types: anxious, avoidant and

disorganized (all considered 'insecure'), and secure. Think of your attachment style as a psychological blueprint that shapes how you connect and relate to others. Everyone – whether single, in a relationship or somewhere in between – falls somewhere along the spectrum of these four styles. Since each style comes with its own patterns of behaviour and needs, it's crucial to understand how different styles complement one another or clash. This knowledge will not only spice up intimacy in your relationships, but your quality of life overall.

Intimate needs when anxiously attached

Those of us who are anxiously attached often feel like our partner isn't as close to us as we'd like. We crave frequent reassurance and validation that we're loved, worthy and safe in our relationships. We want to be close and enjoy lots of affection, whereas distance, separation and unresponsiveness throw us off. This worry can take a toll on our self-esteem. The same thing goes for uncertainty, which feels distinctly unsettling. That's because ambiguity and unresolved issues, especially about where we stand in our relationships, are tough for us to handle. We might feel resentful if we think our partner doesn't fully get us or if we feel underappreciated. We're in tune with our partner's moods and can sense when things are off. However, our sneaky fear of abandonment can make us overthink things and get stuck in loops of catastrophizing, mind-reading and jumping to conclusions (see p. 107). This can lead to unhealthy behaviours and acting out in ways that are jealous, clingy and obsessive.

When it comes to sex, as anxious types we often use it as a tool to ease feelings of not being good enough and the fear of being alone. Sex becomes a way to seek approval, validation and a sense of closeness and security. It's a way to feel whole. We might also use sex to manipulate. We want to be wanted.[6] We might have sex to get attention, to convince someone to commit or to make someone care for us. We tend to fall in love easily and quickly, but our desire for closeness and our fluctuating self-worth also make us more prone to cheating and having sex we don't really want.[7] We're likely to struggle with partners who have avoidant styles, as they find it hard to meet our intimate need for closeness and clarity.

Our challenge with intimacy is to fulfil our need for closeness without compromising our sense of self and pushing away the ones we care about.

Intimate needs when avoidantly attached

On the flip side, those of us with an avoidant attachment style feel like our partners always want to get closer to us and like we're not given enough space. We see this as demanding and intrusive. We value our independence and like to be in control. We're uncomfortable with the idea of having to rely on anyone, or anyone else relying on us. It takes time for us to trust, and we feel skittish and cagey when under pressure from others.

To protect our space, and ultimately ourselves, we

keep an emotional distance from others. We put up a guard, set rigid boundaries and have lots of rules. Even though we may be with someone for years, we don't do relationship talks or contracting (aka agreeing on and setting relationship expectations). We prefer to operate in a grey zone. We use ambiguity as a way of shirking responsibility and as a sort of exit strategy in order to avoid expectations and commitment.

In sex and dating, avoidants like to be with others, but we don't really want to be *together*. We often go for partners who are unavailable, as we subconsciously perceive it as safer that way. Similarly, we also have overly high, if not impossible, expectations of the 'perfect' partner, and we tend to reminisce about a previous one – the so-called phantom ex.[8] As for sex, it's often just physical. It's a thing we do that feels good, a tool for us to unwind, and a way for us to boost our ego.[9] We don't want to want, and so we tend to jump from partner to partner and avoid long-term relationships.[10] That, or we might withdraw from sex and dating altogether. We don't do well with partners with anxious styles, as they find it hard to meet our intimate need for space and ambiguity.

When it comes to intimacy, our challenge is to actually allow it to happen and to have close relationships without pulling away.

Intimate needs when disorganized attached

Last but not least of the insecure attachment styles is the disorganized crew. We're a little less common, and harder to pin down. That's because we're a mix of anxious and avoidant behaviours, making us a bit of a challenge to understand and navigate. A lot of us have had rough starts with abusive upbringings or childhood trauma, where our caregivers were more sources of fear than safety. Those of us with a disorganized attachment style tend to swing back and forth in our relationships, like I did with Calum and Marcus. We crave intimacy, but we're also scared stiff of actually getting it. We long for the same reassurance and validation as the anxious types, but like the avoidants, we're not too keen on the idea of relying on anyone. We reach out for affection and closeness, then suddenly pull back. Our intimate needs can go through big swings, making it tough to keep our relationships steady.

Sex can be just as much of a rollercoaster for us as it is for our partners. Sometimes, like those who are anxiously attached, we might use sex as an attempt to achieve closeness, validation and reassurance. Other times, we might detach from sex, treating it as a purely physical thing. These shifts can lead us to have a chaotic and unsatisfying sex life, where we might oscillate between intensely seeking out sex to feel worthy and engaging in it as an emotionless act. We can find it hard to understand how we truly feel about someone, and are often equally as stumped by our swings as they are.

Our challenge with intimacy is to recognize and learn how to tone down our extremes and bring a bit more stability into our relationships.

Intimate needs when securely attached

Those of us with a secure attachment style, which is about 50 per cent of the population, find it pretty easy to build and maintain relationships.[11] This typically comes from growing up in a stable and nurturing household where relationships were trusting, respectful and supportive. We're comfortable depending on others and being depended on, and we're cool with commitment. In our relationships, we generally feel self-worthy and satisfied, and we don't often act out. We get that different people have different needs, and we don't equate a partner's desire for closeness as a threat to our autonomy, or their desire for space as a lack of love. We can access a wide range of emotions and are able to move through any strong emotions that pop up.

We are able to identify and express our needs, and we encourage our partners to do the same. We view sex as a healthy and integral part of a romantic relationship and a way to build intimacy and enjoy pleasure. We're open to mixing things up in the bedroom, and we enjoy the affection that comes both before and after sex. We're a great pairing for all styles, as we're able to provide solid ground for creating secure relationships.

Our challenge in intimacy is to maintain a healthy balance between the 'push' and 'pull' – especially with a partner who is insecure – and to continue to nurture relationship growth.

PRINCIPLE 4 — CULTIVATE YOUR INTIMACY

Intimacy is a biological need

When we lack intimacy, we risk loneliness. This might seem a bit out there at first, but hear us out. Loneliness is more than the feeling of being alone. It's actually a biological process that kicks in when there's a gap between the social interactions we crave and what we're getting.[12] We're social creatures at heart. Our brains are wired to connect and bond with others. We mirror each other's expressions, regulate each other's blood pressure, and synchronize our breathing and heart rates. Just as we experience hunger and thirst, we all have a drive for social connection.

This drive is influenced by our ability to maintain 'social homeostasis' in our bodies – think of it as your body's way of keeping your social connectivity in balance. You can see this in action when looking at dopamine differences between introverts and extroverts. Dopamine, often referred to as the 'feel good' hormone, plays a role in pleasure, reward and motivation. Here's a fun fact: when hanging out with others, introverts actually get *more* dopamine than extroverts. That is, they feel more satisfied and therefore need to spend less time with others. Extroverts, on the other hand, get *less* dopamine and are therefore driven to seek out more hang-time so they can reach social homeostasis and hit that sweet spot of social satisfaction.[13]

But here's the kicker: when we skimp on social connection, or if we're stuck in a cycle of chronic isolation, it's not only our social life that suffers – our physical and mental health can start to decline too. There's a reason why solitary confinement is such a harsh punishment. The effects of chronic loneliness can increase stress hormones (e.g. adrenaline and cortisol) and lead to all sorts of not-so-great feelings and behaviours, like aggression and irritability, depression, and even becoming less social over time.[14]

Isolation and loneliness can also have a negative effect on our ability to form meaningful bonds and maintain lasting relationships.[15] Remember, you only have one circuit for all types of social bonds. That means the same brain circuitry you used to bond with your caregiver is the same one you use to bond in your adult romantic relationships.

This isn't meant to scare you – it's pretty unlikely you'll find yourself living the life of Tom Hanks in *Cast Away* – but it's crucial to understand how important intimacy and social bonds are for your overall health. Intimacy isn't a luxury or a nice-to-have; it can be a real game changer in warding off loneliness and fostering happier, healthier and more secure relationships. That's why getting clear on what you need from your intimate relationships and building a more secure attachment style, whether with romantic partners or friends, is key. Luckily, we're going to show you how to do just that.

Cultivating intimacy in real life

Whether secure or insecure, the journey to better sex, better relationships and a better life all starts with being

PRINCIPLE 4 — CULTIVATE YOUR INTIMACY

able to identify and express your intimate needs. A big part of this is getting a handle on your attachment style and figuring out how it gels or grates with that of your partner, as well as those of the other people in your life. For instance, if you're on the anxious side, having a secure partner can help to reassure you and soothe your fear of being alone. And if you're more of the avoidant type, a secure partner can give you the breathing room you need without compromising on emotional connection. On the flip side, if you're anxious and you partner up with someone avoidant, it's going to amplify your insecurities; and if you're avoidant and you get with someone anxious, it's going to overwhelm you.

It took me a while (and a lot of work) to move from disorganized to secure, but I did it, and now that I'm here, I'm making sure I do things to cultivate and maintain intimacy. Same goes for Billie. Here's what it looks like in real life for me . . .

Around me, grassy hills rise and fall like a series of gentle waves rolling towards the horizon. I can't remember how many dates Luke and I have been on, but we've been seeing each other for a few months. He's standing at the bottom of the hill, straddling his bike as he waits for me. I zoom down to meet him, sun in my face, wind in my hair, grinning as I get closer. Braking, I pull up next to him. He smiles, dimples forming in his cheeks, and leans over to give me a quick kiss. I catch myself holding my breath and feeling all the lovely warm fuzzies.

'Hey,' he says. Always a man of many words.

'Haiiiiiii!' I reply, giving him another peck and his eyes

sparkle. 'Phew that hill was WILD. I haven't gone that fast in ages! Are you ready?'

'Yeah! You?'

'Mmm, almost.' I pause. 'Have I told you something today?'

He laughs and his smile broadens knowingly. 'No, I don't think you have.'

'Lame. That sucks.' Sticking my tongue out, I push off the pavement and clip back into my pedal. I sprint off in front of him, initiating a race. He curses and I hear the quick click-click of his cycling shoes as he tries to catch up. Both of us are laughing, proper laughs, the ones that come from the belly and make your face hurt from smiling.

'You're such a cheater!' I hear him yell behind me. I feel mischievous, joyful, alive – like I'm connected to myself, to him and to the whole world around me.

'You're sure I haven't told you yet today?' I shout back, still sprinting.

'Definitely sure!' Sun reflects off the river to my right and I swerve to avoid a passing bumblebee. Already hit two of those this summer – wasn't great. I look back to see him gaining on me, less than a metre away.

'I like you!' I feel comfortable and confident saying it, secure in myself and our evolving relationship.

'I like you too,' he shouts back with a grin.

When I look back at how I (failed to) cultivate intimacy before versus how I cultivate it now, the difference is night and day. That late-night ride home in the pouring rain all those years ago was a wake-up call. I realized I had to either work on myself and be around people doing the same, or stay stuck and be okay with that. I was tired of all the recurring arguments, tired of having shit sex and a lack of intimacy, and tired of missing out. I was

PRINCIPLE 4 – CULTIVATE YOUR INTIMACY

neither ready nor willing to settle for a life riddled with dysfunctional relationships.

So, I decided to take a break from dating. As I did, I started to see how my issues with intimacy weren't just showing up in my romantic relationships, but in my other relationships too.

At work, under stress, the anxious part of my disorganized attachment style would kick in and I'd struggle with imposter syndrome and perfectionism, and seek validation from others. I'd wrap my self-worth up in my performance and this belief that if I wasn't 'the best', I wasn't worthy. Then, I'd swing. Stress would make me crave isolation and distance. I would become uneasy about depending on others in my team, because I'd feel like I was no longer in control of my career. I also worried I couldn't rely on them to get stuff done or follow through – it felt like it was all on me.

With friends, I'd swing between seeking closeness and seeking space. I loved spending time with my best friends, but when my self-esteem was low, I'd worry about upsetting them. I'd never say no, and I'd feel responsible for making sure they always had a good time. With new friendships, my avoidant side crept in. Combine that with being an introvert and I was an unstoppable party animal (not). During those periods, I couldn't be bothered to try and I didn't feel like I needed more friends. It took too much energy and too much back-and-forth and compromise. I preferred to do things solo.

My journey to developing a secure attachment style was not a straight path. It came with ups and downs and zigs and zags, but I got there in the end, and now it feels pretty damn good. The real light-bulb moment was learning that attachment styles exist and getting to grips with my own intimate needs. For the first time, I had the words to describe what I was feeling and knew why I was acting the way I was. Turns out, the only thing 'wrong' with me was having a normal reaction to a difficult childhood. Both therapy and coaching helped, and so did connecting with others – and doing a ton of reading and reflecting. But the real breakthrough came when I realized that if I wanted to feel secure, I needed to create security for myself.

I decided to tackle my romantic relationships first, since that's where my emotional swings were most obvious and where I felt most vulnerable. It was also where my experiences with a lack of intimacy or clashes in intimacy were most acute. I dove into 'conscious coupling', which is exactly what it sounds like. Rather than winging it in relationships or falling back into old patterns, I adopted a more intentional approach.

I got more selective about who I was intimate with, how we spent our time, and paid attention to how being with them made me feel – not just during sex, but overall. I kept a list on my phone, giving a thumbs up or thumbs down after a hang. Trust me, seeing a bunch of thumbs down next to someone's name really makes you rethink keeping them around. I started to protect myself from people who made me feel less than or 'blah', and especially those who triggered my unhealthy attachment behaviours. The more I did this, the more I naturally drifted away from people who weren't ready or willing to do the work on themselves.

When I finally opened myself up to more serious dating, it was strange at first. I felt grounded going into it. I'd finally found the 'I' in intimacy and realized I didn't need to search for my other half, because I was already whole. I could clearly and quickly differentiate who was good for me and who wasn't. The weird bit was, when I started dating the ones who were good for me, it felt boring. There was no drama, no emotional rollercoasters; it was ordinary and nice.

PRINCIPLE 4 — CULTIVATE YOUR INTIMACY

Initially, I found the ordinariness a bit unsettling, as if I was missing something. With time, a lot of self-reflection and the help of my therapist, I gradually realized what I was 'missing' was the chaos, and actually I didn't miss it at all. I knew I'd gone through a shift when I developed an appreciation for stability. I started to cherish moments of calm, seeing them not as dull but deeply grounding. If stillness was a love language, it'd 100 per cent be mine. Don't get me wrong, I still want adventure, spontaneity, passion — all that cheesy good stuff — but I've learned not to mistake that for chaos and drama.

Once I'd cultivated a secure attachment style and chosen a partner (Luke) who was secure too, it was all about keeping that going and making space to communicate and respect our intimate needs. We took stock of what intimacy meant to each of us and made lists of what we both needed to feel intimate — with ourselves and with each other. A big one was emotional connection, so we started practising a weekly gratitude ritual, which has since become a lovely habit we have. We also prioritize different types of touch and ensure we have non-sexual touch every day. Last, we combined Luke's need for quality time with my need for shared activities, and have picked up sports and hobbies we can do together. This last one was a fun one because it also gave us the opportunity to bring novelty into our relationship and to see each other through fresh eyes. There's nothing sexier than watching your partner do something they're great at.

One of my biggest learnings along the way has been that cultivating intimacy doesn't mean cutting out dependencies but, rather, finding — and becoming — the right type of person to depend on. I mean, even if we wanted to ditch dependency, it's biologically impossible — we're simply not wired that way. In her book Attachment Theory in Practice, *Dr Sue Johnson explains,*

'From the cradle to the grave, human beings are hardwired to seek not just social contact, but also physical and emotional proximity to special others who are deemed irreplaceable. The longing for a "felt sense" of connection . . . is primary in terms of the hierarchy of human goals and needs.'[16]

*This realization hit me like a ton of bricks: intimacy is more than feeling connected, it's the biological process that **drives** connection. A lack of intimacy isn't just about the feeling of being alone; it has real consequences on our sex lives and our lives in general. From physical health to mental health, from the bedroom to beyond, intimacy is a fundamental part of who we are. I read this quote by Esther Perel and Mary Alice Miller, which sticks with me to this day:*

> *It's been said that we need fifty words in a foreign language in order to speak it. In the language of intimacy, basic fluency comes down to just seven verbs: to ask, to take, to receive, to give, to share, to refuse and to play . . . Verbs are everything we do and everything we do to each other.*[17]

If I want to cultivate intimacy, it's not something that just happens, it's something I need to actively do. I do it by taking, receiving, giving, sharing, refusing and playing. And now, I know how to cultivate intimacy not only with Luke and in my romantic relationship, but across all of my other relationships too.

Whether you're single, casually dating or in a long-term relationship, knowing your attachment style and your needs, as well as those of your partner, not only improves your intimacy but your emotional wellbeing and quality of life overall. So here's the big question: what does intimacy mean to you?

PRINCIPLE 4 – CULTIVATE YOUR INTIMACY

In practice: Here's how to build intimacy IRL

Before you start: Identify and understand your attachment style

Reflect on how you typically behave in your romantic relationships. Answer the questions below honestly and try not to overthink them – there's no right or wrong answer. At the end, tally up your responses to identify your attachment style.* Use our attachment needs 'cheat sheet' (p. 147) as an identification guide and communication resource in your relationships.

ATTACHMENT STYLE QUIZ

1. I am comfortable with depending on my partner and having them depend on me.
    a. Rarely
    b. Sometimes
    c. Often
    d. Almost always
2. I feel confused about my feelings towards my partner.
    a. Rarely
    b. Sometimes

---

* This quiz is designed for self-reflection and is not a definitive assessment. For a more comprehensive understanding of your attachment style, we'd recommend reaching out to a professional and further reading.

c. Often
   d. Almost always
3. I find that my partner's reassurance doesn't ease my worries.
   a. Rarely
   b. Sometimes
   c. Often
   d. Almost always
4. I prefer keeping an emotional distance in my relationships.
   a. Rarely
   b. Sometimes
   c. Often
   d. Almost always
5. I am confident in my partner's love and support.
   a. Rarely
   b. Sometimes
   c. Often
   d. Almost always
6. I feel hesitant to get too close to my partner.
   a. Rarely
   b. Sometimes
   c. Often
   d. Almost always
7. I worry about my partner's commitment to our relationship.
   a. Rarely
   b. Sometimes
   c. Often
   d. Almost always

PRINCIPLE 4 — CULTIVATE YOUR INTIMACY

8. I feel secure and comfortable in my relationships.
   a. Rarely
   b. Sometimes
   c. Often
   d. Almost always
9. I value my independence more than my relationships.
   a. Rarely
   b. Sometimes
   c. Often
   d. Almost always
10. I can rely on my partner when I need help or support.
    a. Rarely
    b. Sometimes
    c. Often
    d. Almost always
11. I find it difficult to fully trust or rely on a partner.
    a. Rarely
    b. Sometimes
    c. Often
    d. Almost always
12. I am comfortable sharing my deepest thoughts and feelings with my partner.
    a. Rarely
    b. Sometimes
    c. Often
    d. Almost always

13. My feelings towards relationships can be inconsistent.
    a. Rarely
    b. Sometimes
    c. Often
    d. Almost always
14. My partner's needs and feelings can overwhelm me.
    a. Rarely
    b. Sometimes
    c. Often
    d. Almost always
15. I find myself clinging to my partner and then pushing them away.
    a. Rarely
    b. Sometimes
    c. Often
    d. Almost always
16. I experience mixed feelings of need and fear in my relationships.
    a. Rarely
    b. Sometimes
    c. Often
    d. Almost always

Anxious style: If you selected 'Often' or 'Almost always' for questions 3, 7, 13, 16.

Avoidant style: If you selected 'Often' or 'Almost always' for questions 4, 6, 9, 14.

Disorganized style: If you selected 'Often' or 'Almost always' for questions 2, 11, 12, 15.

PRINCIPLE 4 — CULTIVATE YOUR INTIMACY

Secure style: If you selected 'Often' or 'Almost always' for questions 1, 5, 8, 10.

Tool #1: Use the attachment needs 'cheat sheet'

BUILDING INTIMACY WITH AN ANXIOUS ATTACHMENT STYLE

An anxious attachment style may mean we feel like our partner is not as close to us as we'd like them to be. Our challenge is to meet our intimate need of closeness while not 'pushing' our partners away. Here are some intimate needs that we might ask of our partners to help us feel more secure:

- **Validate and communicate:** Be consistent with communication and provide validation that we are wanted.
- **Reassure during times of separation:** During periods of physical or emotional separation, provide extra reassurance and time together, face to face.
- **Provide frequent affection and be responsive:** Express affection frequently and be readily accessible and responsive to our concerns.
- **Be clear on commitment:** Avoid ambiguity or uncertainty about our relationship status or its trajectory.
- **Resolve conflict immediately:** Don't delay or leave things unresolved. This makes us more anxious and worsens conflict.

BUILDING INTIMACY WITH AN AVOIDANT ATTACHMENT STYLE

Those of us with an avoidant style may feel like we're not being given enough space and that our partners are trying to get too close. Our challenge is to meet our intimate needs of independence while not overly 'pulling' away from others. Here are some intimate needs that we might ask of our partners to feel more secure:

- **Give space and encourage independence:** We value autonomy, and may feel trapped if we perceive our partner as being too intrusive or demanding.
- **Take it slow with emotional connection:** Let emotional closeness develop gradually so we don't feel skittish.
- **Establish clear boundaries:** Use boundaries to give us a sense of security, autonomy and predictability.
- **Avoid overdependency:** Don't push us for excessive reassurance, and respect our capability to handle things on our own.
- **Recognize our efforts to connect:** Closeness is still important to us, it just looks different.

BUILDING INTIMACY WITH A DISORGANIZED ATTACHMENT STYLE

The disorganized style is less common and often comes from childhood trauma. Those of us with this attachment style oscillate between 'anxious' and 'avoidant' tendencies, displaying mixed signals in our relationships. Our challenge is to minimize these swings, while also providing more predictability for our partners. Here are some intimate needs that we might ask of our partners to feel more secure:

- **Create clarity and predictability:** Provide clear, consistent and predictable behaviour to help us feel less anxious and more open.
- **Reassure in a way that's judgement-free:** Provide a judgement-free space for us to be vulnerable without fear of criticism or rejection.
- **Establish trust:** Give us connection or space when we need it, so we can relearn how to depend on others.
- **Understand it's not about you:** Be patient with us as we heal our internal conflict of desiring intimacy while also fearing it.
- **Help self-regulate:** When we swing, remind us that we are safe and not defined by our past.

BUILDING INTIMACY WITH A SECURE ATTACHMENT STYLE

Those of us with a secure attachment style find it easy to build and maintain relationships. Our challenge is to maintain a healthy balance between the 'push' and 'pull', or to support insecure partners. Here are some intimate needs we might prioritize and build habits around so as to stay secure:

- **Mirror actions and words:** Be comfortable discussing and contracting boundaries and reliable in upholding them.
- **Be emotionally available:** Know and express individual needs, hold space for vulnerability, and share emotional experiences.
- **Have uncomfortable conversations:** Discuss feelings and potentially difficult topics without fear of judgement or criticism.
- **Mutual growth and support:** Set and achieve goals together while also supporting each other to set and achieve goals individually.
- **Enjoy togetherness and separateness:** Normalize spending time and doing activities both together and apart.

Tool #2: Complete an intimate needs inventory

Identifying and expressing our needs can feel like a bit of a puzzle, especially if we haven't taken the time to think about what they are. We've used this exercise a lot with the women we've worked with, to help them dig deeper into their own emotional and relational landscapes. Spend as much or as little time as you need to fill out the prompts below. Remember, this is just for you. The best answer is the honest one – you're going for self-discovery here, which means not hiding from yourself.

We'd also suggest revisiting your intimate needs inventory every few months, to check in on if – and how – your needs have shifted. If you find communication a

PRINCIPLE 4 – CULTIVATE YOUR INTIMACY

bit of a challenge (for you or a partner), this can be a fantastic tool to use as a conversation starter, as well as to explore compatibility and potential areas of conflict. For a downloadable list, go to www.turnyourselfon.co.

MY INTIMATE NEEDS INVENTORY

1. My definition of good sex is . . .
2. My definition of a good relationship is . . .
3. My definition of intimacy is . . .
4. When I'm feeling sad, I need . . .
5. When I'm feeling angry, I need . . .
6. When I'm feeling lonely, I need . . .
7. When I'm feeling tired, I need . . .
8. When I'm feeling ashamed, I need . . .
9. When I'm feeling afraid, I need . . .
10. When I'm feeling stressed, I need . . .
11. When it comes to sex, I'd like my partner to . . .
12. When it comes to money, I'd like my partner to . . .
13. When it comes to family, I'd like my partner to . . .
14. When it comes to helping around the house, I'd like my partner to . . .
15. When it comes to spending time together, I'd like my partner to . . .

Here are some examples from women in our community to help get you started.

Good sex is . . .

- 'A meaningful physical connection with my partner that brings us both pleasure and closeness.'

- *'Feeling really closely connected with your partner, feeling safe and loved, enjoying the moment, and it's pain free.'*
- *'I'm not sure. Sex that I enjoy and my partner enjoys that makes me feel relaxed.'*
- *'Two people sharing each other's bodies, feeling confident and free to enjoy pleasure, resulting in either just enjoying this time together or orgasming together.'*

Your turn . . .

Tool #3: Practise gratitude

When it comes to starting a gratitude practice, we've seen all sorts of reactions. There are the folks who are already onboard, those who are pretty 'meh' about it, and those who think it's a load of fluff. I'll be the first to put my hand up and admit that I used to be in that last group. What we can say is that, despite it sounding a bit 'woo-woo', there's a ton of solid research backing up the benefits of gratitude for relationships, health and wellbeing.[18]

But here's the thing – the real magic of gratitude is in how you do it. Within our neural circuitry, our brains actually get more out of receiving gratitude than giving it. So, while many think of gratitude practices as writing down lists of what we're grateful for, that's not the most effective way to go about it. Instead, you want to create a practice where you receive gratitude, especially in the form of a **story**.[19]

PRINCIPLE 4 — CULTIVATE YOUR INTIMACY

Here are your step-by-step instructions on how to do it:

1. Ask someone you trust (like a partner, family member, friend or colleague) to share 1–3 things about you that they're genuinely grateful for. It's even better if they can ground these things in stories or memories you've shared.
2. Decide how you want to receive their thoughts. It could be written down, spoken out loud, face to face, etc. If you can, have them write their thoughts down and read them to you face to face.
3. While they share, listen actively. Don't interrupt, downplay or deflect. And don't feel like you have to respond or reciprocate right away.
4. Say thank you and genuinely mean it. Appreciate what they've shared and the time they took to do it.

Now, there are two parts of this exercise that might make you squirm a bit. The first is asking someone to say nice things about you, and the second is receiving what they say. If you're feeling hesitant, we'd encourage you to push through it. Growth happens when we step outside of what's familiar and into what's unknown. Reflect on how this exercise makes you feel, and use it to create more opportunities for gratitude on a daily, weekly or monthly basis.

Gratitude is also a fantastic tool for building intimacy with your partner and seeing each other with fresh eyes. Here are some bonus ideas that we've used ourselves as well as with the women we've worked with:

- **Gratitude jar:** Keep a jar in a shared space. Decide how often you'll drop in notes of appreciation about each other. Remember, quality trumps quantity. On special occasions or when the jar is full, sit down together and read them out loud.
- **Nightly gratitude talks:** Before bed, take a minute or two to share one thing you're grateful for about the other person. Focus on actions from that day or week. You can do this in person, via text or over a phone call – whatever works for you.
- **Gratitude letters:** Each month, write a letter to your partner highlighting what you appreciate about them, including stories and moments of connection. Share these letters during a dedicated time, however you'd like.
- **Shared gratitude journal:** Keep a journal where both of you jot down moments of gratitude. This not only creates a collection of positive memories but also provides a space for reflection and conversation.

Look back to look forward

Take 1–2 minutes to reflect and answer the following questions:

1. How am I practising intimacy well?
2. How am I not practising intimacy well?

> 3. What's one action I'm going to start, stop or continue NOW to bring more intimacy into my life?
>
> If you'd like to dive deeper, we've hooked you up with some great resources and downloadable templates at www.turnyourselfon.co.

Cement your learnings

- Intimacy is the process of sharing a bond and feeling connected. It's something you actively do, not just something that happens.
- Intimacy is a two-way street, and a give and take. It's not intimacy if only one person is doing it all.
- When intimacy is missing or you're having issues with intimacy, it can have some pretty big effects on your health and wellbeing, as well as how long and how well your relationships last. We're biologically wired for social connection; it's in our nature to depend on others and for them to depend on us too. It's a valuable thing to nurture, not a luxury reserved for some lucky people.
- There are four main types of attachment style: anxious, avoidant, disorganized and secure. Each style has its own needs, so what feels intimate to you might not feel the same to someone else. That's why it's super important

to figure out and share what your intimate needs are.
- Those with anxious and avoidant styles often bump heads when it comes to intimacy and are more likely to run into relationship troubles. This is because they have opposite intimate needs when it comes to getting close. People with secure attachment styles are usually the best at supporting others and are less likely to set off those insecure attachment behaviours.
- Building and maintaining a secure attachment style is something you have to work on continuously. It means knowing yourself well and being dedicated to regularly cultivating intimacy. Some tools that can help with this include knowing your default attachment style (p. 143), recognizing your own attachment needs (p. 147), creating an intimate needs inventory (p. 150) and practising gratitude (p. 152).

Bonus reads

- Amir Levine, MD, and Rachel Heller, MA, *Attached: The New Science of Adult Attachment and How It Can Help You Find – And Keep – Love*
- Susan M. Johnson, *Attachment Theory in Practice: Emotionally Focused Therapy (EFT) with Individuals, Couples, and Families*
- bell hooks, *The Will to Change: Men, Masculinity and Love*

PRINCIPLE 4 — CULTIVATE YOUR INTIMACY

- Diane Poole Heller, PhD, *The Power of Attachment: How to Create Deep and Lasting Intimate Relationships*
- Robert Karen, PhD, *Becoming Attached: First Relationships and How They Shape Our Capacity to Love*
- Daniel J. Siegel, MD, and Mary Hartzell, MEd, *Parenting from the Inside Out: How a Deeper Self-Understanding Can Help You Raise Children Who Thrive*
- Lindsay C. Gibson, PsyD, *Adult Children of Emotionally Immature Parents: How to Heal from Distant, Rejecting, or Self-Involved Parents*

Principle 5 – Embrace Your Desire

By letting go of what desire isn't, knowing your turn-ons and meeting yourself where you're at

Picture these film scenes . . .

In *Titanic*, Jack and Rose share a sudden steamy moment in the back of a car, with Rose's hand pressed against a foggy window. In *Mr & Mrs Smith*, John and Jane abruptly go from trying to kill each other to a passionate hook-up amid the wreckage of their house. In *Chloe*, Catherine hires Chloe to test her husband's loyalty but finds Chloe's descriptions too hot to handle and ends up in bed with her. And in *Atonement*, Cecilia and Robert's pent-up passion suddenly explodes against a library bookshelf.

And the list goes on . . .

When it comes to desire, we've been fed so many stories about what it's supposed to look like. You know, like two star-crossed lovers from different worlds who accidentally touch and lock eyes for a bit too long, and suddenly there's this uncontrollable and insatiable wanting of each other that leads to the most passionate and mind-blowing sex of their lives.

Let's be real, some of the time it might be like that,

PRINCIPLE 5 — EMBRACE YOUR DESIRE

but most of the time, not so much. In our relationships, desire and sex are often much less spontaneous and steamy than pop culture makes it out to be. There's also this belief that if that 'spark' isn't there or if it fades, something's wrong. That if our relationship is solid, we should be having lots of regular, amazing sex out of the blue. And if we're not, it's a problem and we should resign ourselves to either sexlessness or a 'sufficiently sexual' relationship.[1] Sound familiar?

In the UK, 51 per cent of women have had one or more sexual difficulties in the last year.[2] That means that half of us are struggling with things like lack of desire, feeling anxious or pain during sex, and that figure only includes difficulties that last three months or more. Imagine how much higher that number would be if we took out that time frame. A lot higher. So yeah, sex can feel pretty complicated, and if it does for you, you're not alone.

Low desire is the most common sexual difficulty, and it's something that up to half of all women will experience at some point in their lives.[3] I've been there, Billie's been there, and chances are, we'll be there again. We've also been on both sides of it – the one with more desire and also the one with less. It can be tough, not only on you but on your partner, and on your relationship too. Don't just take it from us though, here are some shares from our community:

- *'I'm feeling deflated, hopeless and not optimistic. It's like, even though I can orgasm, my mind's not in it, it just feels like a reflex. It's like going through the*

motions without feeling the excitement. I'm not sure how to fix it.'
- *'I've tried everything, but nothing seems to work. It's like my desire for sex has just switched off, and I'm worried about what this means for my marriage. I can't help but feel like it's my fault, like there's something wrong with me.'*
- *'I love my partner, but for the past few years, I've had no interest in having sex. I don't look forward to it and I never initiate either. The more I feel like I'm supposed to want sex, the harder it is to actually want it. It feels like more of a chore than anything.'*
- *'I miss the sexual connection we used to have. It's hard feeling like I'm the only one who wants it and like wanting is wrong. I just want us to find a way back to each other again.'*
- *'I try not to take it personally when my partner doesn't seem interested in sex with me, but I worry that I'm not attractive anymore or that I'm not enough. I'm also worried it's going to be like this forever and I'm a bad person for wanting it to be different.'*

Whether you're happy with your level of desire, unhappy, or haven't given it much thought, hello! We've got something for you.

Think of this chapter as the sex ed you needed but probably never got, especially when it comes to understanding desire and how it shows up in your body. Together, we're going to explore why sex is a motivation and not a drive, two different types of desire, and how desire is different from arousal and pleasure. We'll also look at some science on why our minds and bodies don't always feel connected during sex. We'll end by giving you some fun tools to start getting to know your bodies a bit more intimately and to play with touch. When you're done with this chapter, you'll not only know how to embrace your desire and meet it where it's at, but you'll also feel more confident knowing what turns you on, so that you can find your power both in and out of the bedroom.

Desire case study

At some point in our lives, many of us are going to hit a snag in the desire department. We might also find ourselves on the flip side of things, navigating what it feels like to be the one with higher desire. What's interesting is that we don't worry about it all that much when we're alone. It's mainly when we're in relationships, especially long-term ones, that the whole concept of 'having desire' starts to feel like more of a thing. To give you an idea of what this can look like in real life, Billie's got her own story to share.

Billie's story

There were times, like after my assault, where it made sense to me that my sexuality vanished and my desire fizzled out. Other times, like in a loving long-term relationship, I didn't understand it. During these times, I was confused by my loss of desire – I couldn't figure out where it went or how to get it back.

I've already spoken about my first long-term relationship, the one I had with Michael. While I've touched on how my confidence wavered in our relationship, I haven't yet spoken about how my desire fluctuated in it too. This is a story about that. About how I experienced a loss of desire and found myself in a sexless relationship despite being very much in love.

When Michael and I started dating all those years ago, our sex life was 'nice', as the Brits would say. It wasn't super exploratory, but it was fun, respectful and mutually enjoyable. I was focused on my pleasure and on his, and he was the same. We had a great relationship, and a great friendship too. We got on well, had similar interests, and my friends and family adored him. For the first few years, everything felt easy, exciting and right.

Moving to London changed things. Michael was already settled in the city and, confident as he was, had his own routine, life and vision of the future, while I felt like my life was just beginning. That's when I first noticed my desire waning. But it didn't make sense to me at the time, because I still fantasized about other men and had the desire to have sex with myself. It wasn't that I'd lost my desire for sex, it was that I'd lost my desire for sex with Michael.

Living in London made me realize how much more I had to explore. With a new environment and a new job, I felt like Samantha from Sex and the City. I wanted to unleash myself, sexually and otherwise.

That was the first time Michael and I broke up, although we didn't stay broken up for long. The assault hadn't yet happened, I'd still not done the whole building of my self-confidence, self-esteem and self-efficacy thing. Insecurities about my worth and future eventually got the better of me, and Michael and I got back together. He was the safe and familiar option, and I felt silly throwing that away over a lack of desire.

PRINCIPLE 5 — EMBRACE YOUR DESIRE

Then the assault happened and created a domino effect of emotions which impacted my desire and sex life.

The first domino to fall was beginning to feel fear and shame about my sexuality. I blamed it for my assault and began to withdraw from sex altogether because of it. I also never told Michael what had happened; I felt ashamed and guilty, and I couldn't bring myself to talk about it. And so, when it came to having sex with Michael in the aftermath of the assault, it became easier to say no than yes. Instead of confronting the problem, I told myself that I was someone who wasn't all that interested in sex. Because Michael and I weren't comfortable talking about intimacy, we never discussed our desire discrepancies, which meant everything was left unsaid.

Eventually, I lost my desire for sex entirely. The less I was having it, the more it sort of petered out. It seemed easier that way — to accept sexlessness rather than trying to change our relationship as a whole.

In retrospect, when it came to understanding and embracing desire, there was a lot I didn't know. Society had taught me that if I wasn't having 'great sex' all the time, something was wrong. It also taught me that desire should be constant, and that it should be the same throughout the entirety of my relationship, like it was at the beginning. As if how much I desired my partner, and how much they desired me, was a measurement of our relationship's success. If we didn't desire each other, it meant we should just be friends and nothing more. Lastly, society taught me that desire should be spontaneous and passionate — that it shouldn't take work or planning.

As I've shared already, there are many reasons why Michael and I broke up. Of these, our sexlessness and mismatched desire was a major one. I didn't understand what desire was and how it worked, and so ultimately I didn't think our relationship was salvageable or worth saving. Had I known differently, we could have talked about our intimate needs and agreed to work on our sex life together. While we're both very happy with our current partners, our relationship could have had a different ending if we hadn't viewed sexlessness as fatal and if we'd better understood desire – what it is, what it isn't and how it works in practice.

The science: What you need to know about desire

Sex is a motivation, not a drive

First things first, Billie and I are going to share a little bit of science with you that might make you go, 'Wait, what?' – and if we're lucky, may even blow your mind.

There's no such thing as a sex drive: biologically, it doesn't exist.

That's right, just like Billie shared, almost everything we've been taught about desire is wrong.

Let's back up a minute and start with deepening our understanding of biological drives. These are internal states that *drive* us to seek out and perform specific behaviours we need to survive. They're kind of like built-in urges that tell us to do things so we can stay alive. When you're hungry, you know you need to eat. When you're thirsty, you grab a drink of water. When you're tired, you get some sleep. When you're cold, you shiver, when you're hot, you sweat, and when you're

PRINCIPLE 5 — EMBRACE YOUR DESIRE

lonely, you seek out connection – you get the gist. Biological drives are triggered when there's too much or too little of something in our bodies. They're critical to our health because they help our bodies stay in balance (homeostasis), so that we can, quite literally, stay alive.

Here's the thing though. As much as someone might love sex, crave sex or even think they need sex, they're not going to keel over and die without it. Simply put, it's not like food, water or air – it's just not. Think about it. If sex were a biological drive, there's no way we'd be going days, weeks, months or years without it – we'd be in big trouble, to say the least. Plus, as Dr Karen Gurney points out in her book *Mind the Gap: The Truth About Desire and How to Futureproof Your Sex Life*, unlike other biological needs, the less we have sex, the less we actually want it.[4]

Okay, so, we're all on the same page that there's no such thing as 'sex drive'. Where does this concept come from – and why, as a society, are we so hung up on it?

Well, we can thank our old friend Sigmund Freud for that. The (mis-)categorization of sex as a biological drive has its roots in psychological and biological theories that emerged in the 1890s and early 1900s. Back in the day, Freud considered our desire for sex, which he coined 'libido', to be a key drive for survival and procreation.[5] Not surprisingly, there's been a lot of controversy around Freud's work. Apart from the fact that 'libido' varies hugely across individuals – and the whole 'we're not going to die without sex' thing – there's also the point that most of us aren't looking to have a baby every time we get down.

So if our desire to have sex isn't a biological drive, then what *is* it?

Desire is a motivation. It's about wanting sex more than needing it. How motivated we are to seek it out is highly individual and is influenced by a myriad of things way beyond our basic survival.

Sure, some of us might want sex because we're trying to have kids. Most of the time though, we want to have sex because we're seeking pleasure, connection, intimacy, validation and even escapism. For all these reasons – and many more – it makes perfect sense that we're motivated to have sex. We enjoy sex, and want sex, and sex (should) feel great!

Other times, we might *not* want sex. We might be worried about being interrupted, we might feel like we need to shower first or we might be distracted by all the other things we have on. We might be stressed, tired or just disinterested in sex. We might be going through menopause or navigating illness. We might not feel good about ourselves or our body. We might not feel good about our relationship or where it's at. We might not feel good about the sex we're having because it might be unsatisfying or it might hurt. Or, like we saw in Billie's experience, we might not want sex because of power dynamics or because we're afraid or ashamed. There are so many situations and circumstances, all of which are perfectly understandable, in which we might not want sex – and no, it doesn't mean anything is wrong with us or that we're going to die without it.

That's all to say, there's no right amount of sex you should be having. Exactly because sex is a motivation and not a biological drive, there's no fixed range or magic number that dictates whether you're having too little or too much. As Emily Nagoski explains in her book *Come Together: The Science (and Art!) of Creating Lasting Sexual Connections*, the measure for 'great' isn't 'about how much sex you have, but about whether you like the sex you're having'.[6]

Spontaneous versus responsive desire

Now that we know that our desire for sex is a motivation, not a drive, it's time to clear up a second misconception: that desire is spontaneous. Despite what most of us have been taught and what we see in pop culture, there's more than one way to experience desire. Spontaneous desire is the one we're most familiar with: it's when you suddenly – or spontaneously – want sex. You know, that whole 'out of nowhere, a switch gets flicked and you're immediately in the mood' kind of thing.

Now, spontaneous desire is real and many people do experience it. It tends to be more common for men and people with penises, and it's a perfectly normal and healthy way to experience desire. It's just not the only way.

Another perfectly normal and healthy type of desire is responsive desire, a concept introduced by the brilliant Dr Rosemary Basson.[7] This type of desire doesn't pop up out of the blue, but instead emerges in response to something. Think of it as desire that needs a gentle nudge – this nudge being positive sexual stimuli and a sexually appropriate context.[8]

Fun fact: responsive desire is much more common for women and folks with vulvas, as well as in long-term relationships.[9]

Here's an example of what it looks like in action. Imagine you're at home and watching Netflix with your partner, there's no one else around, you've got nothing to do, and you've spent the morning relaxing and hanging out together. At the moment, you're feeling kind of neutral or indifferent towards having sex – you're neither feeling it nor not feeling it. Say your partner starts to massage your shoulders and gives you some nice touches. After a while, the touch, combined with being relaxed at home, starts to make you feel a little frisky and you decide to initiate a make-out. During the make-out, you notice yourself getting turned on. Your original indifference towards having sex shifts towards curiosity and motivation to seek it out: you experience desire.

Whereas spontaneous desire is **desire → arousal**, it's the opposite for responsive desire. Instead, it goes like this: **arousal → desire**. In other words, in responsive desire we want sex in response to something we find sexy, as well as being in an environment that feels good. Likewise, we might not want sex if we find something unsexy and we're in an environment that feels not-so-good, like the power dynamic Billie had with Michael. Now, to understand how responsive desire works on a deeper level, we're going to get a little geeky and talk about your brain.

Remember how in the chapter on self-confidence we said your brain is like a supercomputer designed to take in information and help you make sense of the

PRINCIPLE 5 – EMBRACE YOUR DESIRE

world? Well, within your brain and central nervous system lives a subsystem called the dual control model of sexual response.[10] This is made up of two parts: your sexual excitation system (SES) and your sexual inhibition system (SIS). What makes these parts cool – but also a little tricky – is that they both work independently of one another and also at the same time. In her book *Come As You Are*, Emily Nagoski likens the dual control model to driving a car.[11]

Getting in the mood: Your sexual accelerator and sexual brakes

Your sexual excitation system is like hitting the accelerator. As it scans for sexually relevant stimuli, like the smell of someone's perfume or cologne, and sexually appropriate contexts, like being on vacation, it revs up and tells your body to 'turn on'. A stimulus might be kissing or physical touch, but it can also be things like how you're feeling, your relationship dynamics or the environment you're in. That's because pleasure is personal, and so what gets you going might not be the same as it is for someone else.

Now, while your SES is on the lookout for all that good sexy stuff, your sexual inhibition system is doing the opposite. It's scanning for unsexy stuff and looking out for why you should slow down or stop. From feeling stressed to bad breath to hearing kids next door – like your accelerator, what hits your brakes is individual and can vary a lot from person to person.

The key here is that everyone's accelerator and brakes are different, and so how *sensitive* they are is going to be different too. Some of us might be heavy on the accelerator and barely touch the brakes, while others might be all about the brakes with a less sensitive accelerator. Some of us are somewhere in between. All and any combination is A-okay. Remember, how much we want sex is a motivation, not a drive. That means it's normal for our levels of desire to be different depending on the sensitivity of our accelerator and brakes, as well as whether or not we enjoy the sex we're having.[12]

Which brings us to a common topic for a lot of couples: how to solve desire discrepancy in our relationships. Desire discrepancy is when there are differing levels of desire between partners.[13] Over the last few years, there have been loads of 'women's health' products that have started popping up all over the place, many of which claim to be the miracle cure to 'increase desire'. To save you some time and some money, as well as to avoid potential side effects to your health, we'd like to talk about why many of the 'boost your libido' solutions aren't all that effective.

When it comes to increasing women's desire, you've probably heard all sorts of advice, like 'use a sex toy', 'try a new position', 'watch porn', 'buy lingerie' or even 'take a supplement'. Don't get us wrong, we're all for exploring new things and introducing new practices into your sex life. Toys can be fun, new positions can shake things up in the bedroom, ethical porn can get the accelerator going, and dressing up can make you feel good. As for the supplements – not something we'd

PRINCIPLE 5 — EMBRACE YOUR DESIRE

suggest. They're a bit of a cash grab and there's little to no scientific data showing they actually work, plus the lack of regulation around them is pretty scary.[14]

All that being said, if you or your partner are concerned about low desire, the key thing to remember before you start splurging on stuff is that a lot of these 'libido-boosting' products aren't all that effective. That's because they only focus on hitting the accelerator and don't do much about taking your foot off the brakes. It's also because, when it comes to navigating a desire discrepancy, there's no one-size-fits-all solution, and therefore different strategies need to be applied to different circumstances.[15] To help cultivate desire, especially if it's low, the first step is to experiment with both the accelerator and the brakes, so you and your partner can identify what increases and decreases openness, curiosity and the motivation to have sex. The second step is to talk about one another's accelerator and brakes, and make a plan to find the right balance.

The ingredients you need to enjoy sex

When it comes to enjoying sex, there are two other ingredients you need: arousal and pleasure. Most of us tend to treat them all the same, but they're actually quite different — let's break them down.

By now, you should be a little more familiar with the concept of desire — what it is and what it isn't. If you're nodding in agreement, great!

This next question is for you: What is desire?

If you were able to answer right away, awesome! And

if you weren't, don't worry, here's an answer to help you out.

Desire is 'wanting'. It's a motivation, not a drive, and we can experience it either spontaneously or responsively. Billie and I have a soft spot for pastries, so I'll use an analogy: desire is looking at an almond croissant (or whatever other tasty thing you like to eat) and thinking, 'I've not tried it yet, but hot dang, do I want to eat it.' Desire lights up the brain's reward and motivation centres and dopamine is released, which creates feelings of anticipation and motivation.

One of the things that keeps us wanting is our anticipation of an experience. Sometimes, this can be a pleasurable feeling. We feel curiosity, excitement and optimism. Other times, not so much. Anticipation can make us feel frustrated, anxious and afraid. To quote the brilliant Emily Nagoski again, 'whether desire feels good or not depends on the context'.[16]

Novelty is one way of creating a positive context. It's not just about shaking things up, but also about cultivating desire, especially if you've been with your partner for a while or if things are feeling a little too familiar. In her book *Mating in Captivity: Unlocking Erotic Intelligence*, Esther Perel writes:

> It's not a lack of closeness but too much closeness that impedes desire . . . our need for togetherness exists alongside our need for separateness. One does not exist without the other. With too much distance, there can be no connection. But too much merging eradicates the separateness of two distinct

PRINCIPLE 5 – EMBRACE YOUR DESIRE

individuals ... When people become fused – when two become one – connection can no longer happen. There is no one to connect with. Thus separateness is a precondition for sex: this is the essential paradox of sex and intimacy.[17]

Novelty helps us balance this paradox in our relationships. It's about adding a bit of mystery and surprise back into the mix, letting us see ourselves and our partner as individuals with still more to explore. It's like adding spices to your favourite dish. Sure, the dish is great on its own, but throw in a little pepper, salt and a sprinkle of something unexpected, and you've got a whole new flavour experience. Just as spices can take your meal to the next level, a touch of novelty can make your relationships feel even more exciting.

Desire is different from arousal. If desire is 'I want this', arousal is 'I'm preparing for this'. It's your body's physiological response to sexually relevant information or stimuli, and it's often automatic. It's the physical manifestation of being turned on, like increased heart rate, blood flow, lubrication, genital response, body temperature or that good old fanny-flutter sensation.[18] Back to the croissant analogy, it's taking a bite and having your body respond to it. For instance, your mouth waters, your tummy grumbles and hormones get released. Your body is getting itself ready to eat, digest and do the rest. Arousal kicks off in your autonomic and somatic pathways, activating brain areas like the hypothalamus and amygdala, and releases the hormone and chemical messenger norepinephrine.

And then there's pleasure. If desire is 'wanting' and arousal is 'preparing', pleasure is 'enjoying'. As you eat the croissant, pleasure is the feeling of 'mmmm this tastes so good' as you savour every bite. When something feels pleasurable, your brain's reward centres release neurotransmitters like dopamine, oxytocin (the 'love chemical') and endorphins – your body's natural painkillers. It's like a little party in your brain. We'll do a deep dive into pleasure in chapter 7, but for now, all you need to know is it's about 'enjoying' something.

That's a lot of science we dropped, but it's going to come in handy shortly. If you don't remember all the details, that's okay. Here's a quick tip to help you keep track of what's most important...

QUICK TIP

The main thing you need to remember is that desire is 'wanting', arousal is 'preparing' and pleasure is 'enjoying'.

Arousal non-concordance: When your mind and body are out of sync

Raise your hand if during sex or a sexy activity, you've ever felt like your mind and body weren't in sync?

If so, you're not the only one.

Leading research by Dr Meredith Chivers, a sexologist and clinical psychologist, shows that women

PRINCIPLE 5 – EMBRACE YOUR DESIRE

experience a disconnect between their 'physical arousal' (like wetness) and their mental arousal around 50–60 per cent of the time.[19] This means that in about half of their sexual encounters, how physically turned on a woman is doesn't match how turned on she actually feels in her head. In contrast, for men, this rate is a lot lower, at around 10–20 per cent.

So, what's going on here? What the heck is this disconnect and why are so many of us feeling it?

Let's start with a hypothetical scenario.

Imagine you're reading a book or watching a show, and there's a sneaky little sex scene in it. You might notice that your body starts to get all hot and bothered – getting wet, becoming flushed or experiencing some tingly feels. This is you getting turned on and aroused because your brain has told your body that the sex scene is 'sexually relevant'. But here's where your mind, and how you feel about that sex scene, comes in. Mental arousal happens when a sexy stimulus shifts from being 'sexually relevant' to being 'sexually appealing'.

When both your body and mind agree that something is sexually relevant and sexually appealing, it's called 'arousal concordance'. It's when everything's in sync: you're physically turned on, and mentally you feel it too.

This time, imagine you read or watch that same sex scene, but you're sitting next to one of your family members or a bunch of strangers. Sure, your brain might still see the stimulus as sexually relevant but, given the circumstances, it's no longer sexually appealing. You might have the physical arousal, but mentally you're not feeling it. Your body's physical response and your mind's mental response aren't on the same page. It's like when a song you don't like comes on and your foot automatically starts tapping, even though your mind's not feeling the groove.

This is called 'arousal non-concordance' (or arousal discordance) and it's super common. It can be when the body is a 'no', but the mind is a 'yes'. For instance, you might want to have sex and be really into it, but struggle with vaginal dryness or vaginismus. It can also happen when the body is a 'yes' but the mind is a 'no'. This can be the experience of survivors of sexual violence whose bodies may have gone through physical arousal and physiological responses like lubrication or orgasm during their assault. Just because our bodies react a certain way, it doesn't mean our minds agree. In her book *Better Sex Through Mindfulness*, Dr Lori Brotto explains how many evolutionary psychologists argue that 'this automatic response may have evolved to protect women from infections or trauma during sex'.[20]

Remember how arousal and desire aren't the same thing? That arousal is 'preparing' and desire is 'wanting'? This is where we can see some of their differences playing out in real time. Sometimes you might feel desire without much in the way of physical arousal, or you might be physically aroused but not actually want sex. Sometimes you'll feel both arousal and desire, other times you'll feel neither.

This is one of many reasons why it's important to recognize that consent is not about how aroused we are or aren't, but about how we feel about having sex, and that it is being freely and readily expressed as an enthusiastic 'heck yes!' Equally, as we'll explore in chapter 7, pleasure is so much more than the physiological response of having an orgasm.

Embracing desire in real life

Reflecting on everything you've so far picked up in this chapter, do you see desire in the same way as when you first started reading?

If so, you were way ahead of us! And if not, tell us more — what's changed?

For us, learning what desire is (and isn't) has had a huge impact not only on our sex lives, but on how we feel about ourselves and our relationships too. Instead of seeing desire as an on-off switch or something either you have or you don't, we started to think about it like changing seasons. Here's a look at how that's played out for Billie and how she now embraces desire in real life...

Embracing my desire has involved understanding and accepting that all relationships, including the one with myself, go through seasons. It's about tuning into my desire and recognizing what it feels like in my body. Desire for me is a willingness and deep wanting to have sex with myself and with others. I feel in tune with myself, like all the different parts of me are in sync, and I'm able to access and express my erotic self fully. Sometimes that expression is sexy and powerful whereas other times it's playful and silly.

It's also an incredibly somatic experience where I feel fully present in my body. When I shower for instance, I'll glance at myself in the mirror and I'll turn myself on. I watch myself massage soap on my arms, my hips, my thighs. I feel the hot water tickle my skin as it runs down my breasts. I take in the earthy smell of my shampoo and the whole thing feels incredibly erotic. I become aware of my arousal and the subtle changes going on in my body. My desire becomes a private experience, one that is just for me.

When my desire's low, I equate it with a lack of interest in sex, not only with others but also with myself. I see it as a red flag, a sign that something in my life needs attention. Instead of viewing it as a flaw in my relationship, like something is 'broken', I see it as an opportunity for self-exploration and discovery.

For example, I now know that power dynamics are crucial to shaping my desire and that feeling powerless really hits my brakes. I mentioned earlier that I have had two major long-term relationships in my life, my ex Michael, and the wonderful Seb. Seb is my current partner and we've so far been together for seven years. From day one, we were equals, both in and out of the bedroom. It's one of the things that attracted me to him so much in the first place. Throughout our relationship, we have always had open and honest conversations about sex, decision-making and how to honour and respect each other's needs.

Don't get me wrong, we've experienced all seasons of desire, from one of us wanting more sex than the other, to periods of mutual low desire. What sets this relationship apart is that we recognize these shifts and talk about them. Depending on whether we're in the same season or not, we adapt our sex life to meet both of our needs.

When our desires are mismatched, for example during a season where his desire is higher than mine, we will discuss our accelerators and our brakes and agree to put some practices in place to

PRINCIPLE 5 — EMBRACE YOUR DESIRE

create opportunities for intimacy. I enjoy massage, which works as a sort of 'jump start' to turning me on. We decided to schedule that on a weekly basis but made sure that we agreed that there was no expectation of sex that came along with it.

We also believe in taking responsibility for our own desire. When one of us is in a higher-desire season, we're open about it, and the other supports them in self-care. So for instance, when my desire is higher, I'll lean into my erotic fantasies, watch some Erika Lust and enjoy a lovely little midday masturbation, without guilt or shame. (Side note: Erika Lust is an award-winning filmmaker who creates ethical, relatable and sex-positive adult films, which are beautiful by the way. If you haven't seen her work, I highly recommend it!)

When we're in different seasons, we still find ways to connect, whether that's through having a massage or a cuddle, taking a shower together, or even a bit of finger, hand or oral play. We both understand there are loads of different things we can do to create a sense of closeness and connection other than having S-E-X. Whatever season we're in, Seb and I move through them together.

With my previous partner Michael, I lacked the tools (and the self-esteem) to address our desire discrepancies. I withdrew from physical and sexual intimacy altogether because I didn't want to accidentally do something that would lead him to initiate. I also now get how it feels to be on the other side of things, where you think you need to sacrifice your needs so as not to be disrespectful or put pressure on your partner.

The biggest steps in embracing my desire have been understanding and accepting it, unlearning and relearning what desire means for me, and educating my partner too. I've learned it's normal for desire to ebb and flow, and I now know how to create an environment that nurtures my desire and my relationship. Embracing desire is not about waiting for spontaneity but about cultivating a space where my partner and I can both thrive.

In case you need to hear it again (and even if you don't): it's normal for desire to go through seasons. If you're in a high season, that's okay. If you're in a low season, that's also okay. And if you're in shoulder seasons, guess what – that's okay too.

Desire is a motivation, not a necessity. Sex is something we want, not something we need, and sometimes we want it, and sometimes we don't. There's more than one way to experience desire. For some, it might be spontaneous, but for many of us, it's responsive, which means creating an environment – mentally, emotionally and physically – that enables you to feel open and curious about sex. This is why it's so important to get to know your accelerator and brakes and to discuss them with your partner. While desire is important to cultivating great sex, it's not the most important thing. What makes sex great isn't how much you have it or how much you want to have it, it's whether it feels pleasurable when you do.

In practice: Here's how to embrace your desire

Tool #1: Create a desire inventory

Creating a desire inventory is like making a cheat sheet for what turns you on and what turns you off, in and out

PRINCIPLE 5 — EMBRACE YOUR DESIRE

of the bedroom. It's a way to look at your desire from all angles and get you thinking about what revs you up and what slows you down.

The goal is to fill out the table on the following page and come up with a plan to make sure your sexual experiences — whether solo or with someone else — are tailored to what you need. Sharing this with a partner can be a game changer. It opens up a conversation about what each of you is into and helps you find common ground where your turn-ons and turn-offs might clash.

To kick things off, we've included examples from Billie on the next page . . .

If you'd like a downloadable version, head over to www.turnyourselfon.co.

Tool #2: Practise body mapping

Body mapping is a tool that helps you connect with your body, identify your boundaries and explore your turn-ons (and -offs) through the power of your own touch. It's super easy to get caught up in the hustle and bustle of life, juggling a million things and falling into the same old routine. That doesn't leave much room for self-care or self-discovery, which also doesn't leave much room for cultivating desire. This practice is like hitting the pause button on all that noise. It's a chance to (re)discover your own body and connect to your sensual self. Body mapping is also about mapping what feels good for you and tapping into your inner erotic guide.

Category	My turn-ons	My turn-offs	Actions I can take
Physical Stimuli			
Touch	Cuddling, firm massage, the feeling of water on my skin...	Touching my belly after I eat or when I feel full...	Tell Seb that my desire for sex is lower after big meals...
Tastes	Chocolate, freshly brushed teeth, kissing after Seb's eaten something sweet...	Kissing after Seb drinks coffee or when I haven't brushed my teeth...	Brush our teeth before sexy time and carry mints on date nights out...
Sights	Seb's big beaming smile, warm natural light, sexy lingerie...	A dirty bathroom, harsh artificial lighting...	Dress up for myself and send Seb a cheeky pic....
Sounds	Quietness, ocean waves, a crackling fire, Beyoncé...	Hearing Seb's niece and nephew next door...	Make a playlist of songs that make me feel sexy...

Smells	Fresh laundry, the sea breeze, lavender, earthy candles, Seb's cologne...	Smelling like BO (like after the gym), the smell of beer on Seb's beard...	Take a shower together and use it as a form of foreplay...
Emotional stimuli	A balance of power, feeling equal in my relationship, feeling connected...	Feeling unworthy or like my value is tied to being good in bed...	Maintain equality in my relationship and introduce power play...
Intellectual stimuli	Deep conversations and debates about topics I'm interested in, good banter...	Positions on topics that go against my values, misogyny...	Start a couples' book club with Seb....
Environmental stimuli	Outdoors, a little bit of risk like being caught, voyeurism, in the mornings...	Being at my parents' house when my family is home....	Wake up 15–30 minutes earlier so Seb and I can have a cuddle...

Here are your step-by-step instructions for body mapping:

1. **Create a sensual space:** Find a private, comfortable area where you can lie down and explore without interruptions. Set the mood with soft lighting, some chill tunes or a bit of white noise, lock the door if you can, and do anything else that helps you take your foot off your brakes.
2. **Get comfortable:** Undress however much you'd like and lie down or lean back in a supported position. With your eyes open in a soft gaze, take five deep breaths in through your nose and out through your mouth. Feel your body begin to arrive.
3. **Do a five-senses meditation:** Start to wake your senses up by tuning into each of them. What are five things you can see? Four things you can feel? Three things you can hear? Two things you can smell? And one thing you can taste?
4. **Flex and relax:** If you feel comfortable, close your eyes. Beginning at your feet, flex them for 5–10 seconds and release. Moving your way up to your head, continue to tense and relax different body parts and muscle groups. Feel the weight of your body as an anchor.
5. **Imagine getting a massage:** You can feel warm, skilled hands gliding over your skin, releasing tension from your head down to your toes.

PRINCIPLE 5 — EMBRACE YOUR DESIRE

   a. Where do you want to be touched? Where don't you want to be touched? Where do you want to be touched but only in certain circumstances?
   b. What types of touch do you want? Do you want slow/fast, firm/light or long/short strokes?
   c. Now, imagine that it's someone sexy giving you a massage. How, if at all, would you want it to be different?
6. **Explore self-touch:** Start to touch different parts of your body, exploring various pressures, speeds and motions. Notice how your skin responds to different types of touch like light strokes, firmer pressure, circular motions, pinching, etc. Touch your head, face, ears, neck, shoulders, arms, hands, chest, belly, hips, legs, feet, and anywhere else you feel a sense of wanting.
7. **Focus on your genitals:** If you have a vulva, use your fingers (and some lube if you like) to explore it. Start by placing the whole of your palm and cupping between your legs. Notice the temperature and any textures. Try tracing your inner and outer labia and sandwiching your clitoris between the two. Experiment with circling, tapping, flicking and zig-zagging your clitoris. Move to the opening of your vagina and circle it a few times; if you like, experiment by sliding one or two fingers inside of yourself and notice the different textures.

a. How comfortable do you feel with self-touch? Are there any areas you don't want to touch or explore? Are there any areas you're curious to explore more of?
b. What, if any, sensations felt interesting? What, if any, sensations were you not interested in?

8. **Reflect on your boundaries:** As you continue to explore your whole body, think about your boundaries. If anything feels uncomfortable, pause and reflect on that sensation. Likewise, if anything feels good, do the same. This awareness will help you communicate your boundaries and express your sexual needs.

9. **Conclude with gratitude:** Finish your practice by expressing gratitude to your body for its capacity for pleasure. Take a few deep breaths, gently stretch, and slowly come back into the space around you.

10. **Make your body map:** You can do this by either drawing an outline of your body (front and back) or writing a list. Mark down:
    a. Green – spots that you enjoyed having touched
    b. Amber – spots that you're curious about having touched or are open to having touched but only in certain circumstances
    c. Red – spots you don't want touched (for now or for ever)
    d. If you can, add the types of touch you'd like too. Think about pressure, pace, motion, etc.

PRINCIPLE 5 — EMBRACE YOUR DESIRE

11. **Share your body map (optional):** Whether it's a casual partner or a long-term one, we'd recommend using your body map as a conversation starter. It's a great way to practise setting boundaries, expressing yourself, and leaning into your power.

Tool #3: Make a touch menu

When it comes to touch, one way of balancing our accelerator and our brakes is knowing what types of touch we want and how we want it. The solution? A touch menu. A touch menu can be done solo or partnered, and it's all about exploring different types of touch both in and out of the bedroom. Not only is this a great tool for building intimacy, it also helps with communication so that you can confidently ask for what you want, when you want.

Some examples of types of touch to explore (feel free to add any others)...

- Formal touch: Touch in a public or more formal setting
- Friendly touch: Touch in an informal or more casual setting
- Comforting touch: Touch you'd give for support, soothing or reassurance
- Affectionate touch: Touch that lets someone know you like and care about them
- Playful touch: Touch that is silly, goofy or teasing

- Sensual touch: Touch that is erotic but not necessarily sexual, like a head massage
- Sexual touch: Touch that's intended for sexual pleasure
- Aggressive touch: Touch during conflict or when angry
  - Note: do not act this one out. Instead, discuss it and chat about what you and your partner consider inappropriate and disrespectful (e.g. pulling away, turning your back on the other person, slamming doors, etc.)

IF PARTNERED . . .

With your partner, go through the list of types of touch above, and experiment with each one for two minutes. During which you'll do the following:

- For each type of touch, you and your partner will take a one-minute turn being the 'giver' and a one-minute turn being the 'receiver'.
- The giver's role is to ask, 'What are your boundaries?' and to give the type of touch the receiver asks for, making sure to check in and get feedback.
- The receiver's role is to state their boundaries and to ask for where and how they'd like to be touched.
- At the end, spend 1–2 minutes discussing each type of touch. For example, what you liked,

PRINCIPLE 5 — EMBRACE YOUR DESIRE

kind of liked, didn't like, and what you learned about yourself or the other person.
- Make sure to agree ahead of time on a 'no sex' rule for this exercise. The reason being, when we take sex off the table, it can be easier to focus on enjoying the present moment rather than where the moment is 'headed'. It's also a great way of building anticipation and bringing a bit of erotic tension into your play.

IF SOLO . . .

You'll imagine these types of touch, and feel free to act them out on yourself too. When you're done, write down how you'd like to give/receive them in a list.

Look back to look forward

Take 1–2 minutes to reflect and answer the following questions:

1. How am I embracing my desire well?
2. How am I not embracing my desire well?
3. What's one action I'm going to start, stop or continue NOW to better embrace desire in my life?

If you'd like to dive deeper, we've hooked you up with some great resources and downloadable templates at www.turnyourselfon.co.

Cement your learnings

- Sex is a motivation, not a drive. There's no magic number that dictates whether you're having too much or too little sex. It's normal to want sex you enjoy and it's also normal not to want sex you don't enjoy.
- Desire can be spontaneous or responsive. Responsive desire is more common for people with vulvas. It's not desire that pops up out of the blue, but instead emerges in response to positive sexual stimuli and a sexually appropriate context.
- You have a sexual accelerator and sexual brakes. They both work at the same time and are independent of one another. Your accelerator is all the sexy stuff that turns you on and your brakes are all the not-so-sexy-stuff that turns you off. Desire comes from hitting the accelerator, while also being sure to take your foot off the brakes.
- Arousal is 'preparing', desire is 'wanting' and pleasure is 'enjoying'.
- Sometimes our minds and bodies feel out of sync during sex. This happens when they don't agree on what's sexually relevant and sexually appealing. The mind might say yes but the body says no, or the mind might say no but the body says yes. We call this arousal non-concordance and it is

normal, and solvable by working through the above.

Bonus reads

- Angela Chen, *Ace: What Asexuality Reveals about Desire, Society, and the Meaning of Sex*
- Lori A. Brotto, PhD, *Better Sex Through Mindfulness: How Women Can Cultivate Desire*
- Emily Nagoski, PhD, *Come As You Are: The Surprising New Science That Will Transform Your Sex Life*
- Dr Karen Gurney, *How Not to Let Having Kids Ruin Your Sex Life: Navigating the Parenting Years with Your Relationship Intact*
- Esther Perel, *Mating in Captivity: Unlocking Erotic Intelligence*
- Dr Karen Gurney, *Mind the Gap: The Truth about Desire and How to Futureproof Your Sex Life*
- Sherronda J. Brown, *Refusing Compulsory Sexuality: A Black Asexual Lens on Our Sex-Obsessed Culture*

Principle 6 – Honour Your Health

By understanding your body, taking time to rest and rediscovering play

'Sex is better when I want it and enjoy it' – do you agree or disagree?

Let's assume most of us agree and we're aiming for sex that we're both interested in having and that also feels good. Pretty straightforward? It should be, and yet at no other point in human history have we been so busy – never have our lives been so full and yet so unfulfilling.[1]

Here's a 'fun' fact: over the last year, a whopping 74 per cent of Brits were so stressed that they were overwhelmed or unable to cope.[2] And it's not only stress we're up against either. During our lifetimes, one in three of us will navigate an anxiety disorder and/or depression,[3] with that figure being even higher for folks in the LGBTQIA+ community.[4]

Right about now, you might be asking yourself: what's all this got to do with sex?

Two main reasons. First, as we discussed in the previous chapter, sex is a 'nice to have' (i.e. a motivation) not a biological 'must have' (i.e. a drive). Second,

PRINCIPLE 6 – HONOUR YOUR HEALTH

for many of us, desire is not spontaneous but responsive. For these two reasons, what's going on outside of the bedroom can have a major impact on what's going on inside it. After all, it's not like the moment we walk through our bedroom door, our mind suddenly switches off and our body hits a giant 'relax and reset' button, although it would be awesome if they did.

There's much research – especially that of women's sexual health experts Dr Lori Brotto, Dr Rosemary Basson and Dr Meredith Chivers – exploring the link between low desire, sexual functioning and mental health.[5] For example, in her book *Better Sex Through Mindfulness*, Dr Brotto reveals that there's a 75 per cent chance your desire will drop if you're experiencing depression.[6] When you think about it, this makes sense. When life's got you juggling a million things, jumping from one to-do to the next, and you're running on empty, your sex life may well find itself taking a back seat.

It might even be the case for you that just the thought of stopping, of stillness or of taking time to care for yourself can make you feel stressed. As if it's another thing, right up there next to 'have more sex', that you need to add to your never-ending to-do list. If that's the case for you, here's a gentle nudge to let you know you should be hitting pause right about now – for your sexual wellbeing, and your overall wellbeing too. After all, it's a lot easier for you (and a relationship) to stop before you hit a breaking point rather than becoming a hot mess and needing to put all the pieces back together again.

Think of this chapter as a good friend who's checking in on you. We're going to explore some of the biology underpinning your central nervous system and how mental health can impact your sex life. Plus, we'll explore the importance of rest for both your sex life and your overall health, and how play can be a form of 'pleasure-care' for you and your relationships. By the end, you'll have a better understanding of what's happening in your body, know how to hit the pause button, and have discovered what kind of play brings you energy, both in sex and in life.

(Not) honouring your health case study

Before you read this case study, we'd like you to do a little self check-in. Close your eyes if you can and take a quick moment to reflect on your overall health right now. Think about things like sleep, diet, exercise, mindfulness, community, stress, screen time – also juggling kids if you have them . . .

Ask yourself: 'Over the past month, how have I been feeling?'

On a scale from 1 to 10, with 1 being 'I'm basically a walking zombie' and 10 being 'I'm the poster child for health and wellness', where do you land?

Now, think about your sex life. Would improving any aspects of your health give it a boost? For example, catching up on sleep, getting more regular movement or taking a holiday? What, if any, areas of your health could use a little more TLC?

PRINCIPLE 6 – HONOUR YOUR HEALTH

Full disclosure, the first time I did this reflection, I thought I was acing it.

As you're about to see, it turned out I wasn't . . .

Now, you might be thinking, 'Yeah, yeah, self-care, got it.' Or maybe you're already a pro, and if that's the case, we'd love to hear your secrets. Wherever you fall on the taking-care-of-yourself spectrum, consider my experience a cautionary tale of what can happen when you don't listen to your body and you neglect to honour your health.

Anna's story

Imagine your lungs being crushed and crumpled like an empty paper bag, stuck together, like they just won't fill. You can't breathe, it feels like you're choking, but there is nothing there. You gulp at the air but you can't pull enough down. Heat floods your body, making its way upwards, pooling around your chest and your neck. Your face is on fire. It's too hot, you're too hot. You rip off your jacket and throw it on the ground. You open your eyes and the bathroom stalls around you start to bend. Your vision tunnels. The tiled floor stretches away from you as if it is being pulled into a black hole. You drop to your knees, disoriented and dizzy.

When you try to stand back up, you're shaking so badly that your legs can't hold your weight and they buckle beneath you. Crying, you lie down on your side and curl up in a ball, tucking yourself underneath the rows of sinks on the bathroom floor of the coffee shop. You squeeze your knees into your chest and scrunch your eyes shut. The tiles feel cold against your burning skin. Your teeth start to chatter violently. The rapid, rattling sound of enamel on enamel hammers in your head. Your tongue and fingers prickle.

They feel as if they are being poked by a hundred tiny tacks. A tingling sensation fills your mouth. You're going to be sick. Rolling onto your hands and knees, you crawl towards one of the stalls and start dry-heaving. All the muscles in your torso go rigid, straining against retching wave after retching wave. The only reprieve is in the momentary suffocation of each dry heave.

You start to sob. You hear the noise of it, but you don't recognize it as your own. It sounds like grief and terror — loud, ragged, detached. You've sweated through your shirt, wet dark circles spreading beneath your armpits. But you're cold, freezing cold. The hair on your arms stands straight up, your skin covered in goosebumps. You can't stop shaking. You can't remember when or even how you got here. Time is skewed and your sense of place distorts. You look at your hands and you don't recognize them as your own. A new wave of panic hits you and you suddenly feel claustrophobic in your own body. It's like you're wearing someone else's skin and none of this is real. You aren't real. You gulp at the air once more, but you can't pull enough down.

It starts all over again.

This is what I experienced on and off every day for months. I was in an acute state of survival, getting hit by panic attack after panic attack. I'll say it straight up: sex was the furthest thing from my mind. With everything I was feeling, all I could think about was getting through it, and sex didn't register as a priority whatsoever.

In losing the last reserves in my body, I lost my sense of self — and alongside it, not only my interest in sex but in dating and relationships altogether. I couldn't stand to be in my body or with my own thoughts, let alone share them intimately with someone else. I was stuck. I no longer recognized who I was. I'd spent decades being a perfectionist and a chronic people-pleaser, always *trying to be 'better' and never setting boundaries or saying no. I didn't even know I had trauma – let alone big 'T' trauma (and lots of it). I felt overwhelmed by all the things I had to do and the expectations I had to meet – sexually, romantically, personally, professionally and societally. I felt like I was drowning and I could barely get my head above water to stay afloat, let alone swim to shore. I was being pulled under by the weight of it all and I was both terrified and exhausted.*

At the same time, I felt nothing.

I was trapped in a deep apathy and a total disinterest in everything and everyone. I withdrew from life, from love and from sex. I lost track of time and went from feeling like a minute took forever to suddenly realizing that hours, days and weeks had slipped by. I lost my desire and enjoyment not just of sex, but of life. It was like I was moving from one moment to the next, all on autopilot – like I was there, but not really there.

Alongside feelings of depression, there were also feelings of anxiety and panic, which brought with them a chronic sense of worry and fear, making me terrified of being alone with my thoughts. And so, to avoid overthinking, even though I had no interest in sex or dating, I found myself aimlessly going out with people I wasn't interested in, simply to escape my own mind.

During the few times I did end up having sex, it wasn't pleasurable at all – I neither wanted it nor enjoyed it. It was as if I were floating outside of my body, watching myself go through the motions and performance of sex, but I wasn't actually present while I had it. I knew something was wrong, but I couldn't put my finger on what that something was. As my mental health deteriorated, I found myself going round and round in circles in all areas of my life, and my sex and dating life all but ceased to exist. I oscillated between feeling so acutely present in my body that it quite literally made me sick, to feeling disassociated and detached from it, like I was an alien living in someone else's skin.

At the beginning of 2018, as I was finishing my DPhil, reeling from an unexpected bereavement and starting Ferly, everything came to a screeching halt.

My body had finally had enough. I'd been pushing it too hard for way too long. I'd been failing to take care of myself, never letting myself rest or recover, and I'd also lost my sense of play. In the words of my therapist, I was in the midst of a 'fabulous mental health breakdown'. I'd been headed there for a while, years actually, but I didn't have the knowledge or language to understand the signs. The worst of it lasted about three months, most of which I don't remember. It's a blacked-out gap in my head with scattered images, like a redacted report of my own life. I lost 1.5 stone in six weeks, was running on 3–4 hours of sleep a night and banking about 4–5 panic attacks a day.

In addition to therapy, I was on a hearty dose of sleeping pills, antidepressants, beta blockers and Diazepam, plus Omeprazole to protect my stomach from all the post-panic-attack dry vomiting. It seemed like everything I'd been avoiding in my life had finally caught up with me. The official diagnosis was major depressive disorder, general anxiety disorder, panic disorder and complex post-traumatic stress disorder. There was also a dash of burnout (which wasn't actually an 'official condition', so apparently didn't count).

So, yeah . . . try putting that on Bumble.

It was in the depths of despair about my brokenness that I realized no one else – and certainly not the random men I'd been dating – could fix me; it was up to me. Yes, I needed the help of my close friends and family, but if I wanted to find my way back to life, I couldn't keep lingering on my brokenness. In hindsight,

PRINCIPLE 6 – HONOUR YOUR HEALTH

that's the joy of being broken though – you get to choose how to put yourself back together again. In the end, I became my own kintsugi – through rest and recovery, I was able to mend myself and to heal.*

The science: What you need to know about honouring your health

So here's the thing: if you truly want to have great sex, and you want to have it on a regular basis (whatever 'regular' means to you), you need to honour your health and take care of yourself. There's no way around it. While this is true for everyone, it's even more important for those of us who experience responsive desire (see p. 167). As you saw in my story, when life gets real, sex – and our interest in having it – is often one of the first things to go.

Now, if you're reading this book, you're probably someone who already understands the importance of health and taking care of yourself. What you might be less familiar with is what taking care of yourself looks like inside your body and how not taking care of yourself can impact your sex life.

---

* Kintsugi is a Japanese art form where broken pottery is repaired with gold or other precious metals. Instead of hiding the cracks, kintsugi highlights them, turning them into beautiful lines that enhance an object's beauty. This technique symbolizes embracing flaws and imperfections as part of an object's history, creating something unique and valuable.

So, we're going to put our science hats on and take a high-level look at your autonomic nervous system.

You know how your pupils get bigger or smaller depending on how much light is in a room? Or how your heart races when you're scared? Or how you breathe when you're asleep?

That's your autonomic nervous system (ANS). It controls and regulates a lot of the processes going on in your body so you don't have to think about them. Your ANS is basically your body's conductor, keeping involuntary functions like your heart rate, digestion and breathing playing in perfect sync so you don't have to direct them yourself.

Within your ANS are your sympathetic ('be alert') and parasympathetic ('be chill') systems. Together, they're a sort of scale, constantly adjusting to create a beautifully balanced equilibrium or homeostasis in your body.

Ever heard of the expression 'fight or flight'?

That's the sympathetic ('be alert') nervous system kicking in.

It's your body's call to spring into action and enter a state of hyperarousal. When in hyperarousal, your heart beats faster and pumps blood to your muscles. Your pupils dilate and let in more light. Your breathing quickens to take in more oxygen, and if you're anything like me, you start to sweat hard to keep yourself cool. That's all topped off with a tasty shot of adrenaline, which gives you a kick to tackle whatever stressor you're facing.

But, like an athlete needs rest, your sympathetic nervous system does too.

PRINCIPLE 6 – HONOUR YOUR HEALTH

Without it, your body will stay in a state of hyper-arousal and you'll struggle with things like sleep, digestion and hypervigilance – this is when you're continuously on the lookout for (perceived) signs of danger. As you saw in my story, when this system is chronically activated, you're also less likely to want sex, as your body is operating in 'survival' mode and it's not as much of a priority as keeping you safe and getting your body back to a healthy baseline. This is why we often see a drop in desire with things like chronic stress and anxiety, which activate our sympathetic nervous system and push us into a state of hyperarousal.

Instead of living in survival mode, we need to make sure our ANS switches off and our parasympathetic ('be chill') system kicks in. The parasympathetic system is like your body's cool-down phase after a workout. It's the deep breath, overhead stretch and slowing heart rate that soothes your nerves and helps you 'rest and digest'. It is also the sweet spot to be in if you want to be more open to sex, as well as increase your desire, pleasure and chances of orgasm. That's because you're operating from a calm and relaxed place of 'thriving' rather than 'surviving'.

When your nervous system is balanced, it's like a well-oiled machine, ready to not only help you want and enjoy sex more, but also handle whatever life throws your way. On the flip side, when your nervous system is out of whack, it can take a serious toll on both your sex life and your life overall. This is where the connection between sex and mental health comes in.

Sex and mental health

While it might not be a connection you'd think to make right away, mental health and sexual wellbeing are like two peas in a pod. Whether it's feeling more connected to ourselves and our partner, having the energy and the enthusiasm to initiate sex, or giving ourselves permission to find pleasure in the present moment, when our mental health is good, we feel good. And when we feel good, we're more open to sex and to all the enjoyable experiences that can come with it.

Equally, when our mental health is not so good, it's pretty standard for sex to become less of a priority. This is why you might find yourself experiencing a lack of interest in sex or a loss of desire. Likewise, if you're struggling with your mental health, what happens during sex might change too. For example, you might find yourself ruminating or feeling anxious, disconnecting and detaching from your body, experiencing pain or discomfort, or having difficulties with lubrication and/or orgasm.[7]

That's because conditions like stress act as the body's own personal alarm system, encouraging it to respond to things that the brain perceives as a threat. This could be anything from trying to meet a looming deadline, fighting the flu or even having sex. It's basically your body's way of looking out for you.

Now, a little stress here and there isn't necessarily a bad thing. Good stress, or 'eustress', can actually be a benefit. Like how being exposed to germs can improve

PRINCIPLE 6 – HONOUR YOUR HEALTH

your immune system or how jumping in a cold lake can wake you up and improve your ability to self-regulate.[8] Your sympathetic nervous system kicks in, and once the stressor has passed, the parasympathetic nervous system takes over – allowing your body to chill out and return to its normal baseline.

But here's the thing: your body is built for sprints, not never-ending marathons. When the worry that accompanies stress becomes out of proportion to what's actually going on – that's anxiety. It's like your alarm system is glitching, sending out 'Danger!' signals even though you might not be under threat. Whether it's in your daily life or your sex life, you might become irritable, feel a sense of dread or even experience anxiety and panic attacks.[9] And let me tell you, these are about as fun as trying to afford a house in the current economy.

In addition to the impacts of stress and anxiety on our mental health and sex lives, there's also depression. Instead of constant worrying, depression is more a deep, persistent sadness or lack of interest in life – and yes, you guessed it, in sex too.[10] One of the biggest impacts of depression on our sex lives – beyond this loss of desire – is a loss of pleasure. This is called 'anhedonia' and it influences our ability to enjoy sex. It's like going from living life in rainbows (shout out to Radiohead) to nothing but a dreary grey. Depression also increases the risk of developing a sexual dysfunction by 50–70 per cent. The reverse also holds true: if you have a sexual dysfunction, you're 130–210 per cent more at risk of developing depression.[11] So yes, the two are very much connected.

And then there's trauma . . .

Given that a whopping 70 per cent of us will experience at least one traumatic event in our lifetime, it's fair to say that trauma is real and can have a profound impact on our lives, especially when it comes to sex.[12]

Dr Paul Conti, in his book *Trauma: The Invisible Epidemic*, describes trauma as something that causes emotional and/or physical pain and leaves a lasting mark on a person and their life going forward.[13] Despite common misconceptions, it's not just a bad memory; it's something that physiologically alters the brain and body. In *The Body Keeps the Score*, Dr Bessel van der Kolk writes: 'After trauma, the world is experienced with a different nervous system. The survivor's energy now becomes focused on suppressing inner chaos, at the expense of spontaneous involvement in their lives.'[14]

Similarly, Dr Peter Levine, in *Waking the Tiger*, explains: 'We tense in readiness, brace in fear, and freeze and collapse in helpless terror. When the mind's protective reaction to overwhelm returns to normal, the body's response is also meant to normalize after the event. When this restorative process is thwarted, the effects of trauma become fixated and the person becomes traumatized.'[15]

Given that trauma can manifest in a whole suite of physical ways, from fibromyalgia to chronic fatigue to autoimmune diseases, it's no wonder it can also have a major impact on our sex lives. Even more so for those of us who are survivors of sexual violence.

The unfortunate reality is that while many of us want sex to be a place of play, exploration and pleasure, the lasting impacts of trauma – whether sexual or otherwise – can make sex difficult to enjoy, especially given that it's such an intimate experience.

Because the traumatized brain is often on high alert and scanning for danger, trauma can make it hard to trust others and to be vulnerable with partners. This also makes it tough to relax and connect. Like we saw with the attachment styles in chapter 4, for trauma survivors, sex and intimacy can feel like a bit of a minefield, triggering memories of past experiences or unconscious fears.

In romantic relationships, trauma can also show up as re-enactment patterns, where without even realizing it, survivors end up in relationships that are eerily similar to those in their past where trauma occurred. Subconsciously, this is a way for us to try to 'fix' the past by replaying it and trying to understand it, so we can experience a different outcome. But, instead of helping, it can make things feel way more complicated and chaotic, especially in the bedroom.

In order to move through trauma – as well as stress, anxiety and depression – we need our dysregulated nervous systems to regulate themselves. That means teaching our bodies that we're not under threat, and it's safe to authentically connect with ourselves and with others, not just between the sheets but in the wider world around us.

A sexual recharge: The power of rest

In order to allow our nervous systems to regulate, which also allows us to be in a position where we're more open to sex, we need to learn how to actually rest.

Rest is all about hitting pause on life's constant hustle so you can let your parasympathetic system take over. While sleep is super important, rest is about more than catching some zzzs – rest is both an action (to rest) and a state (being rested).[16] It encourages you to recharge and reset so you can get back to – and maintain – your fullest self, both in and out of the bedroom.

Rest is not a luxury and it doesn't have to be complicated. As Audre Lorde writes in *A Burst of Light* when she talks about her own self-care while fighting cancer and advocating civil rights:

> I had to examine, in my dreams as well as in my immune-function tests, the devastating effects of overextension. Overextending myself is not stretching myself. I had to accept how difficult it is to monitor the difference . . . Caring for myself is not self-indulgence, it is self-preservation, and that is an act of political warfare.[17]

So, in case you need to hear it: rest isn't indulgent and it's not idleness. Rest is what allows us to show up as the most sustainable version of us – for ourselves, our partners and our communities. Rest is also the thing that's going to give us the greatest odds of creating the ultimate sex life we're striving for. It's essential not only to our health and wellbeing, but to our survival, and we need it – a lot of it.

Forty-two per cent of our time, actually.[18]

That's right, according to science, 42 per cent of our day is meant to be spent resting. Now, assuming you're aiming for the designated 7–9 hours of sleep (and yes, that includes you, parents), that leaves a minimum of 1–3 hours of rest in your day.[19] Emily and Amelia Nagoski put it brilliantly in their book *Burnout*: 'If you don't take the 42 per cent, the 42 per cent will take you. It will grab you by the face, shove you to the ground, put its foot on your chest, and declare itself the victor.'[20]

And yet, many of us don't take the rest we need. That's because some of us think we can power through without it, while others deny it for ourselves, and some of us don't have the privilege to access it easily.

Unfortunately, when we do try to 'rest', we often don't. We zone out in front of the TV, scroll through social media, get drunk, maybe crush a king-size Cadbury's Dairy Milk bar. As for sex? Think about how so many of us masturbate. We put our vibrators on max, maybe watch some porn, and orgasm as quickly and efficiently as possible. We do everything we can to avoid slowing down, being still and facing boredom – or, god forbid, being 'lazy'. Instead of resting, we distract and we numb.

Dr Anna Lembke, in her book *Dopamine Nation*, talks about how modern life is filled with distractions that help us escape everyday stressors and emotions.[21] While these distractions provide temporary relief, they also contribute to feelings of disconnection and dissatisfaction. Similarly, numbing behaviours, often used to cope with emotional pain, leave us detached from our feelings and experiences – and that includes sex. It's no wonder so many of us are struggling with things like cultivating intimacy, getting in the mood and having an orgasm.

TURN YOURSELF ON

THIS *IS NOT* WHAT RESTING LOOKS LIKE

Here are some examples of distracting and numbing behaviours (and no, these do not count as rest).

Distracting behaviours include . . .

- **Overworking:** It's like we're on a treadmill, running faster and faster, trying to outrun our own thoughts and feelings.
- **Excessive screen time:** Scrolling and binge-watching becomes our shield, protecting us from facing what's going on inside.
- **Overplanning:** We pack our calendars so tight that there's no room left for introspection or dealing with our emotions.
- **Shopping:** Retail therapy becomes our go-to, hoping that a new purchase will fill the emotional void.
- **Compulsive sexual activity:** We use sex as a distraction, keeping our minds busy so we don't have to face what's bothering us.
- **Sexual risk-taking:** We chase thrills, using the adrenaline rush to drown out our emotional pain or boredom.

And here are some examples of numbing behaviours . . .

- **Overeating:** Food becomes our comfort blanket, smothering our emotions.

PRINCIPLE 6 – HONOUR YOUR HEALTH

- **Substance abuse:** We turn to alcohol, drugs or nicotine, hoping to blur the sharp edges of our feelings.
- **Excessive gaming:** Video games become our escape pod, transporting us to a world where our emotions can't reach us.
- **Avoidance:** We become masters of evasion, dodging social interactions and responsibilities that might force us to confront our feelings.
- **Emotional isolation:** We build walls around ourselves, choosing solitude over the risk of emotional exposure.
- **Pornography overuse:** We retreat into a world of fantasy, seeking refuge from reality and our emotional discomfort.

THIS *IS* WHAT RESTING
LOOKS LIKE . . .

Now that you know what distracting and numbing behaviours look like, here are some ways you can actually rest and honour your health. Keep in mind these are suggestions to help you make informed choices, and this is by no means a definitive list . . .

- **Sleeping:** Aim for 7–9 hours (or as much as you can); avoid bright lights; avoid eating three hours before bedtime; make your room cold; take a hot shower or bath before bed; use white noise.

- **Viewing daylight:** Get at least 10–15 minutes of natural daylight within the first hour of waking (30 minutes if cloudy).
- **Unplugging:** Set aside 30–60 minutes per day to disconnect from all of your devices and the noise of the online world, and tune into the natural sounds around you.
- **Eating mindfully:** Choose one meal a day for this, and as you eat, pay attention to what you touch, see, smell, taste and hear. Notice what hunger and fullness feel like.
- **Getting movement:** Aim for at least 150 minutes of low-intensity exercise per week. Think brisk walking, yoga, easy swimming or gentle cycling.
- **Connecting IRL:** Spend at least three hours of quality time (in person) with people who give you energy during the week, to reduce feelings of loneliness or isolation.
- **Ditching alcohol:** There are many medically backed reasons to cut down on booze. We might love our G&Ts, but the reality is that alcohol wreaks havoc on our bodies.
- **Creating cool stuff:** Tap into your creative side, whether it's through painting, writing, colouring, playing music or whatever else gets your creative juices flowing.
- **Self-pleasuring:** Forget about a vibrator (or try dialling it down). Set a timer and spend 10–20 minutes enjoying your own self-touch without all the extra stimuli.

PRINCIPLE 6 – HONOUR YOUR HEALTH

- **Having a cuddle:** This one's pretty self-explanatory. The only thing to add is if you're worried about desire discrepancies, make it clear it's only a cuddle and not sex.

> **QUICK TIP**
>
> Instead of overwhelming yourself by trying to do it all, start by picking one thing to focus on. Whether it's something you do daily, weekly or even monthly, make it realistic and achievable. Once you've made a habit out of it, move on to the next thing. The goal is to create behaviours that last, so take it one step at a time. And hey, if there are other activities that allow you to rest, reset and recharge, add those to your list too!

Pleasure-care and the importance of play

Honouring our health isn't only about rest, it's also about finding the joy in life and experiencing activities that bring us pleasure.

Sigh. Remember the good old days of building forts and playing hide-and-seek? When we used to do things because they were fun and felt good? When we used to not get so caught up in adulting and being responsible, productive or efficient? When we used to let ourselves *play*?

It might sound slightly out there to suggest that

playing – and letting go and giving yourself permission to feel free – is a productive thing to do. This is especially true for those of us who've been led to believe that being a 'responsible adult' is practically synonymous with getting work done and being busy. Arguably, the responsible thing to do is to actually take care of yourself, which means making rest and play a regular part of your routine.

In fact, one of the most pleasurable ways of recharging our batteries is doing exactly that: playing – and yes, this can include sexy play too.

In his book *Play*, Dr Stuart Brown talks about play as more a state of mind than an actual activity: 'Play, for me, [is] the essence of freedom. The things that most tie you down or constrain you – the need to be practical, to follow established rules, to please others, to make good use of time, all wrapped up in a self-conscious guilt – are eliminated. Play is its own reward, its own reason for being.'[22]

Like sex, play doesn't have a purpose, and that's the whole point – it's just for fun. Play is something you choose to do because it feels good, not because you have to. Also, like sex, play can be purely for your pleasure. That's because sex is a form of play – one that lets you forget about time and get lost in the moment. One that gives you the chance to shed self-consciousness, be present in your body and exist in a state of flow. One that encourages you to improvise and to discover new ways of thinking, doing and being.

Play, which can include solo and partnered sex, is a form of what we call 'pleasure-care'. Pleasure-care is when you recognize and prioritize pleasurable practices and activities that enhance your overall wellbeing and quality of life. Just as you need to rest to honour your health, you also need to play. Indeed, it's through play that you can unlock your full potential for pleasure and weave the many magical moments of joy into your life, both in and out of the bedroom.

Your play personality and types of play

Like sex, what turns each of us on and brings us pleasure in play is personal.[23] According to Dr Brown, we each have a dominant play personality (and typically one or two minor types), which become even more pronounced as we get older.[24] These are:

- **The Joker:** Loves a bit of mischief, a good laugh and being silly.
- **The Kinesthete:** Gets a kick out of moving, grooving and using their bodies.
- **The Explorer:** Thrives on discovering new things and going into the unknown.
- **The Competitor:** Gets pumped up by the challenge of winning.
- **The Director:** Enjoys planning, calling the shots and organizing experiences.
- **The Artist/Creator:** Finds joy in making and creating things.
- **The Collector:** Hunts for cool objects or experiences to find and share.
- **The Storyteller:** Revels in weaving tales and using imagination.

Sure, as adults, play can feel a bit indulgent, but like rest, it's not. It's legit a part of who we are. It's a chance for us to regulate our nervous system, improve our mental health and experience pleasure in our everyday. In her blog, Esther Perel hits the nail on the head:

> Sure, we can engage in play as adults because it's healthy, because it releases endorphins, and so on. But that's kind of like saying that one should have sex because it burns calories. Just like sex, playing as adults is about pleasure, connection, creativity, fantasy – all the juicy parts of life we savour.[25]

We're hardwired to play – it's literally built into the survival centres of our brains.[26] That's because play is important for our cognitive and social development; it's not just recreational but something that helps us to learn and bond. As grown-ups, even though we might write it off, play is still crucial for our happiness, creativity and wellbeing. Not only can it help regulate our emotions and reduce stress, it also lets us bring fun into our romantic relationships and maintain a richer and more satisfying sex life.[27]

A big part of play is social bonding.[28] And without play, we can get a little territorial, possessive and aggressive in our relationships – we are animals, after all.[29] Play keeps the balance, letting us tackle tough times with a wink and a smile – and maybe even a cheeky bum-grab. It's our chance to get creative with our partners, be a little naughty and explore the lighter and less serious side of ourselves.

Through a lifetime of research, Dr Stuart Brown has

PRINCIPLE 6 — HONOUR YOUR HEALTH

identified seven different ways we tend to play.[30] Based on his research, we've come up with some of our own suggestions on how you can be more playful in the bedroom (without it necessarily being all about sex):

- **Attunement play:** This is all about connecting with your partner, like when you lock eyes, share a secret smile and whisper sweet nothings (or shout them nice and loud).
- **Body play and movement:** Turn your bedroom into a sensual playground with things like acro-yoga, a relaxing massage or a cheeky striptease.
- **Rough-and-tumble play:** Ever had a playful wrestle in bed? That's rough-and-tumble play at its best. It's a way to let off steam, enjoy a bit of power play and connect through physicality.
- **Object and sensory play:** This could be running an ice cube over your partner's chest, playing with a vibrator or other toys, or licking warm chocolate off your partner's lips.
- **Social play:** Double dates or group activities are a way to bond with your partner while connecting with others. Looking for something more? Discuss and explore options like consensual non-monogamy, sex parties, voyeurism, swinging and group sex.
- **Imaginative play:** Think role play and costume play, whether that's pretending to be strangers, secret agents or dressing up in

lingerie. Experiment with different sides of your erotic selves.
- **Storytelling and narrative play:** It's not just for bedtime stories. Try writing yourself erotica, sharing fantasies with your partner or sexting throughout the day.

> ### QUICK TIP
>
> In daily life, knowing your play personality and that of your friends, family and partner is a great way to think about how you structure quality time together. Remember that what feels fun for you might not be as fun for others, so it's a cool way of balancing out activities.
>
> In the bedroom, make sure to incorporate play that suits both your play personality and that of your partner. Switch it up by using different types of play, like object play, movement play or a bit of rough and tumble. Who knows – it might be the injection of fun you're craving.

Honouring your health in practice

We all know how crucial it is to take care of ourselves, yet somehow it often ends up on the back-burner. When it comes to enjoying sex that we genuinely want, it won't happen if our nervous system is out of whack or if

PRINCIPLE 6 – HONOUR YOUR HEALTH

we're not in the right headspace. Recovery from my own breakdown didn't happen overnight – and neither did bouncing back in the bedroom. But making it through the darkest period I've ever known opened my eyes to the true meaning of honouring my health and just how vital rest and play are across all aspects of our lives.

Here's a glimpse into what that recovery journey looked like for me . . .

The first thing I did was stop. Not because I wanted to, but because my mind and body were like, 'Nope, that's it, girl,' and then they staged a full-on rebellion. In the beginning, all I could do was survive. Legit. I'd been so busy with overworking, overtraining and, well, over-everything-ing, that I'd missed the warning signs my body had been sending me.

I'd tricked myself into believing that I'd been taking care of myself because I was going to the gym and eating well. While I knew mental health was important, as it turned out, I wasn't doing all that much to maintain it.

Needless to say, when you're trying to survive, your sex life goes to shit. That's because when your mental health is hanging by a thread, the last thing on your mind is having sex. It's also tough to feel sexy when you're tired and all you want to do is sleep. And let's be real, going on Bumble in the midst of a mental breakdown wasn't the healthiest behaviour. It was the ultimate distraction, and neither the sex nor the dates went well for anyone involved.

Acknowledging I was a hot mess was easy – when you're hyperventilating on the floors of public bathrooms, it's pretty hard to deny it. Accepting it was harder. I was broken and there wasn't an easy fix. I needed help. Luckily, I had some great humans who loved me, showed up for me and became my lifeline. Around the same time, I also started therapy, which was long overdue.

The first way I started to take care of myself was by getting rest, and specifically by prioritizing sleep. That being said, it's hard to sleep when you're worried about not being able to sleep, especially when you know how important it is.

So, I got into the nap game.

I napped at home, I napped at friends' houses, I napped at work. Some might have even called me the Nap Master. If koalas could talk, they would have been calling me for tips. They'd have to leave a voicemail though because, you guessed it, I'd be napping.

Alongside sleep, everyone was telling me that I needed to rest.

Rest, rest, rest.

But other than sleeping, I didn't actually know how to rest, or maybe it was more that I couldn't. I hated sitting there thinking about all the stuff I had to do and how much time I was wasting by sitting there 'resting'. So, instead of resting, I'd distract myself. I went through three seasons of RuPaul's Drag Race *and rewatched all of* Buffy the Vampire Slayer. *None of it made me feel rested though – if anything, I felt even more drained (and then guilty for not being rested).*

For me, I had to learn that rest didn't mean vegging out, it meant relaxing, and that rest could also be active. I started doing gentle things that helped me recharge. I rediscovered my love of fantasy and sci-fi books, which allowed me to wander the streets of Imre and sand-walk across the dunes of Arrakis, all from the cosy comfort of home. I also started stretching, practising meditation and doing breathwork. These practices helped me quiet the noise in my head, and learn how to sit with the scary sensations in my body but not be overwhelmed by them. Honouring my health meant giving myself permission not only to rest, but also to heal and recover.

PRINCIPLE 6 – HONOUR YOUR HEALTH

Once I'd moved through the most acute stages of my recovery, and my nervous system began to balance itself out again, I became aware that something in me was missing, or rather something had been lost. I wasn't quite sure when, or where, or even how – all I knew for certain was that it had gone. It wasn't a sudden thing, not like randomly losing a sock. It was more gradual, like losing your favourite book. It used to be right by your bed, then on your shelf, and then in a box as it moved with you from place to place. Years later, you find yourself chatting with a friend and you offer to let them borrow it. But when you go to grab it, thinking it's tucked away somewhere, you realize it's gone. You search all the usual spots, convinced it's just misplaced, but it dawns on you – without even noticing, you've lost it.

It was like that.

Somewhere along the way, I'd lost my sense of joy and my ability to play.

It was like being in the film Pleasantville *(before Joan Allen discovers masturbation and has an orgasm in the bath). I felt like I was walking around in greyscale when the world was meant to be experienced in colour. Honouring my health didn't only mean resting, but also rediscovering how to let go, be free and have fun – how to play.*

Through a process of trial and error, I started to relearn how to play as an adult. At first it was awkward and forced, and I felt guilty and self-conscious and like I should be using my time better. See that cognitive distortion and 'should' creeping in there?

At the time, I didn't yet know about the different play personalities, but I did figure out that I loved to play in ways that let me explore and learn new things, as well as ways that encouraged me to move and use my body. I also liked being silly. I adventured into new territory that combined the different aspects of play I enjoyed – swimming, dancing, rock climbing, longboarding and boxing. With these types of play, I was getting a two- (and even three)-for-one type of deal. I took care of myself by trying new activities, moving my body and building communities, where I could dip in and dip out, in ways that felt good for me.

At the same time that I was exploring play outside of the bedroom, I also began to discover play inside it – starting with solo play.

In the place that I was living, my closet door had a full-length mirror on it. Uncomfortable and awkward as hell, I challenged myself to use the mirror as a tool for mindful play, where I could explore and reawaken my dormant sexuality. It became a way for me to learn how to let go, to feel free and to observe and appreciate my body without judgement or shame. I'd have a bath, put some sexy music on and lock my door. In front of the mirror, I'd play with myself through touch, breath and movement. I'd look at the way my back arched as I rocked my hips, the way my chest rose and fell as I inhaled and exhaled, and the tightening of my muscles as I tensed. I'd watch the graceful curve of my neck as I leaned my head back, and listen to the faint, breathy sounds that slipped out from my lips as I shut my eyes and self-pleasured.

I wasn't yet ready to play with partners again. Not because of any reason other than the fact that I was enjoying my own company and finding peace and joy in being alone but not lonely. Together, rest and play allowed me to take care of myself and to improve my mental health. After having spent way too long hiding in the dark, I was finally able to light myself back up from the inside.

When our nervous systems are out of balance, it throws a wrench in pretty much every area of our lives, sex

PRINCIPLE 6 – HONOUR YOUR HEALTH

included. If you're juggling loads of stress, it's normal for your sex life to get bumped down the list. That's because sex is a motivation, not a drive. So, when you're feeling drained or exhausted, in the battle between sex and sleep, sleep often comes out on top – it's a biological necessity, after all.

It's easy to push ourselves too hard because, well, we can. But just because we can push it, doesn't mean we should. Trust us, preventing a breakdown is much more manageable than recovering from one. Honouring your health means nurturing your whole self – not just your body but your mental and emotional wellbeing too. That means tuning into what your body tells you, taking the rest you need and finding your playful side. This will help you find and ignite your spark in all areas of your life.

In practice: Here's how to honour your health

Tool #1: Do some breathwork

Breathwork is a secret weapon that can help you switch from a high-alert mode to a more relaxed, rest-and-digest state. Beyond the fact that it's been practised for thousands of years, there's also a lot of great science to back it up.[31] Breathwork is all about using different breathing techniques to help regulate your nervous system and bring your body back to a state of equilibrium. We've included a few different types of breathing below for you to play with. Give these a go whenever you need a little reset.

Box breathing:

1. Sit or lie down comfortably.
2. Inhale slowly through your nose for a count of four.
3. Hold your breath for a count of four.
4. Exhale slowly through your mouth for a count of four.
5. Hold your breath again for a count of four.
6. Repeat for 1–5 minutes.

4-7-8 breathing:

1. Sit or lie down in a comfy spot.
2. Inhale slowly through your nose for a count of four.
3. Hold your breath for a count of seven.
4. Exhale forcefully through your mouth, making a *whoosh* sound, for a count of eight.
5. Repeat for 1–5 minutes.

Physiological sigh:

1. Find a comfy spot to sit or stand.
2. Take a deep inhale through your nose, and add a little more air with a second quick inhale.
3. Exhale slowly through your mouth.
4. Repeat for 1–5 minutes.

PRINCIPLE 6 — HONOUR YOUR HEALTH

Alternate nostril breathing:

1. Sit comfortably with your spine straight.
2. Use your right thumb to close your right nostril.
3. Inhale slowly and deeply through your left nostril.
4. Close your left nostril with your right ring finger, then release your right nostril and exhale.
5. Inhale through your right nostril, close it with your thumb, release your left nostril and exhale.
6. Repeat for 1–5 minutes.

Tool #2: Try progressive muscle relaxation

When you're feeling stressed, your body naturally tenses up. It's like your muscles are getting ready to spring into action. This is all part of your sympathetic nervous system, which is super useful if you're facing a real threat but not so much when you're worrying about everyday stuff. That's where muscle relaxation techniques, like the tense-and-release practice, come in handy.[32] By intentionally tensing and relaxing your muscles, you send a signal to your brain that it's time to chill out. This can help turn down the volume on the 'alert' response and activate your body's relaxation response instead.

Here are your step-by-step instructions:

1. **Find your happy place:** Get comfy in a quiet spot where you can chill without distractions. You can lie down, or sit in a cosy chair.
2. **Breathe and settle in:** Take a few deep breaths in through your nose and out through

your mouth (or try some of the breathwork techniques above). Let your body anchor itself with each exhale.

3. **Start at your toes:** Focus on your feet. Tense them up as much as you can – imagine you're trying to scrunch up a towel with your toes. Hold for a few seconds, then let go and relax. Feel the tension melting away.

4. **Work your way up:** Move to your calves. Tense them up, hold, and then release. Notice how it feels when you let go. Keep going up your body, moving to your thighs, hips, belly, chest, arms, hands, shoulders, neck and face. Tense each part, hold, then release. It's like you're going on a little tour of your body, giving each part a moment to shine and relax.

5. **Keep breathing and enjoy:** Once you've worked through your whole body, take a few deep breaths. Feel how much more relaxed your body is now. It's like hitting the reset button.

6. **Check in with yourself:** Take a moment to notice how you feel overall. If there's any spot that still feels a bit tense, give it another go. It's all about listening to your body and giving it what it needs.

Tool #3: Uncover your adult play personality

As you now know, we all have our own unique way of having fun and letting loose. Inspired by Dr Brown's eight play personalities, we've designed this exercise to

PRINCIPLE 6 – HONOUR YOUR HEALTH

help you uncover, explore and articulate your preferences and styles of play within your intimate relationships.[33] By reflecting on different aspects of play and how they manifest in your life, you can gain insights into what brings you joy and fulfilment in the bedroom and life in general. Are you the Joker who's all about the laughs, the Kinesthete who loves to move or maybe the Creator who's always crafting cool stuff? What about your partner? Let's find out...

PART I: REFLECT

1. Grab something to write with or somewhere to take notes, and find yourself a place to journal where you won't be distracted.
2. Take some time to answer the following questions:
   - When you were a kid, what did you like to do for fun? What didn't you like doing?
   - Can you recall a time when you felt particularly playful or free? Where were you, who were you with and what were you doing?
   - As an adult, when you want to relax or have fun, what are your go-to activities? (Tip: focus on the activities you want to do, not ones you think you should do.)
   - What kind of activities do you find most enjoyable when spending quality time with your friends or your partner? What don't you enjoy?
   - What does 'play' in a relationship look like to you? What are examples of behaviours you think are playful?

3. Now look back through your answers. What do you notice? Take a moment to reflect on any common themes and consider which types of play resonate the most with you.

PART II: IDENTIFY YOUR PLAY PERSONALITIES AND FAVOURITE PLAY STYLES

Based on your answers to the questions above, go through the following two lists and put a tick next to the statements that most resonate with you. Limit yourself to a maximum of three ticks per list. For extra fun, feel free to invite your partner to do the same.

Play personalities

- __ **The Joker:** You love to make people laugh and find humour in everyday situations.
- __ **The Kinesthete:** Movement and physical activity are your go-to forms of play.
- __ **The Explorer:** You're curious about the world and love discovering new things.
- __ **The Competitor:** You enjoy games and challenges and always strive to win.
- __ **The Director:** You love organizing activities and taking the lead in group settings.
- __ **The Collector:** You take pleasure in gathering and categorizing objects or experiences.
- __ **The Artist/Creator:** You express yourself creatively through various mediums.

PRINCIPLE 6 – HONOUR YOUR HEALTH

__ **The Storyteller:** You have a rich imagination and love creating and sharing stories.

Types of play

__ **Attunement play:** Connecting emotionally, like a meaningful conversation over dinner.
__ **Body and movement play:** Engaging in physical activities, like dancing or swimming.
__ **Rough-and-tumble play:** Playful physical contact, like play-fighting or wrestling.
__ **Object and sensory play:** Exploring through touch and creation, such as cooking or crafting.
__ **Social play:** Interacting in group settings, like playing board games or team events.
__ **Imaginative play:** Engaging in creative make-believe, like fancy dress or role-playing games.
__ **Storytelling:** Crafting stories, like blogging, podcasting or sharing at social gatherings.

PART III: PUT IT INTO PRACTICE

Now that you've uncovered your dominant play personalities and the types of play you enjoy, think about how to put them into practice.

- How can you incorporate these playful elements more consciously into your life and your intimate relationships? Are there new ways of playing that you'd like to explore with your partner?

- Reflect on any barriers that might prevent you from embracing play. How might you overcome these?

End your journaling session by summarizing the key insights gained and any actions you plan to take.

A LITTLE BONUS LIST FROM US . . .

Here are some ideas for how to experiment with your play personalities in the bedroom, across different play styles:

- **The Joker:** Build anticipation by teasing your partner during sexy play; laugh during sex; get cheeky and mischievous by doing something (consensually) naughty.
- **The Kinesthete:** Explore different sensations with feathers, ice or massage oils; engage in a sensual dance or a playful wrestling match.
- **The Explorer:** Experiment with new positions, props or types of touch; discover each other's erogenous zones with a blindfolded game.
- **The Competitor:** Have a playful competition to see who can resist temptation longer; create a sexy scavenger hunt with rewards for each find.
- **The Director:** Plan a themed romantic evening or a fantasy role-play night; take turns directing each other's touch during partnered masturbation.
- **The Collector:** Create a collection of intimate memories, like love notes or photographs;

collect and use different types of lingerie or toys for variety.
- **The Artist/Creator:** Paint each other's bodies; do a boudoir photoshoot; craft a homemade sex toy or piece of erotic art together.
- **The Storyteller:** Share your fantasies and create a story together; write a steamy short story or love letter for each other; exchange sexts and let it build throughout the week.

Look back to look forward

Take 1–2 minutes to reflect and answer the following questions:

1. How am I honouring my health well?
2. How am I not honouring my health well?
3. What's one action I'm going to start, stop or continue NOW to honour my health going forward?

If you'd like to dive deeper, we've hooked you up with some great resources and downloadable templates at www.turnyourselfon.co.

Cement your learnings

- Your health and wellbeing affect everything in your life, including your sex life. It's all connected.

- Your autonomic nervous system (ANS) is like the behind-the-scenes manager for your body, taking care of all the stuff you don't need to think about. It's got two modes: sympathetic ('alert mode') and parasympathetic ('chill mode').
- When your sympathetic nervous system is activated, your body is focused on tackling a stressor and keeping you alive, so when you're in this state, it's pretty common for sex to be pushed to the back-burner. Same goes for when you're navigating conditions like stress, anxiety, depression and trauma. If your mental health is suffering, your sexual wellbeing and sex life are likely to suffer too.
- In order to create a rich and satisfying sex life, you need to be able to regulate your nervous system and allow the parasympathetic system to kick in. This allows you to be in a position where you're interested and able to enjoy sex. Two powerful tools for doing this are rest (see pp. 205–211) and play (see pp. 211–216).

Bonus reads

- Gabor Maté, MD, *When the Body Says No: The Cost of Hidden Stress*
- Emily Nagoski, PhD, and Amelia Nagoski, DMA, *Burnout: The Secret to Unlocking the Stress Cycle*

PRINCIPLE 6 – HONOUR YOUR HEALTH

- David D. Burns, MD, *When Panic Attacks: The New, Drug-Free Anxiety Therapy That Can Change Your Life*
- Johann Hari, *Lost Connections: Uncovering the Real Causes of Depression – and the Unexpected Solutions*
- Bessel van der Kolk, MD, *The Body Keeps the Score: Brain, Mind, and Body in the Healing of Trauma*
- Paul Conti, MD, *Trauma: The Invisible Epidemic: How Trauma Works and How We Can Heal From It*
- Gabor Maté, MD, and Daniel Maté, *The Myth of Normal: Trauma, Illness and Healing in a Toxic Culture*
- Natalie Y. Gutiérrez, LMFT, and Jennifer Mullan, PsyD, *The Pain We Carry: Healing from Complex PTSD for People of Color*
- Pooja Lakshmin, MD, *Real Self-Care: A Transformative Programme for Redefining Wellness*
- Stuart Brown, MD, with Christopher Vaughan, *Play: How It Shapes the Brain, Opens the Imagination and Invigorates the Soul*

Principle 7 – Prioritize Your Pleasure

By exploring eroticism, tuning into your senses and leaning into your imagination

Just as we've been fed stories about what our desire is 'supposed' to look like, we've also been told what pleasure in sex is 'supposed' to be: the big O. For fun, Billie and I googled 'orgasm' and stumbled upon a treasure trove of headlines promising how to have mind-blowing, toe-curling and out-of-this-world orgasms.[1] Beyond creating FOMO of the incredible orgasms you're 'missing out on', there are also a ton of articles about how to have multiple orgasms, because 'one is never enough'.[2] And as if that's not enough pressure, we should also be optimizing our orgasms, so that we can climax more quickly but make it last longer. But here's the kicker: apparently, it's all 'easier than you think'.[3]

Our culture's obsession with orgasms puts a heck of a lot of pressure on us, our partners and the sex we're having. It's why we get so many shares like these:

- *'I get frustrated because sex seems to finish when my husband finishes and I'm still left wanting more.'*

PRINCIPLE 7 – PRIORITIZE YOUR PLEASURE

- *'I'm turning 50 soon and still I have never had an orgasm. I feel like I'm missing out on something big, like "great sex" is a party I'll never be invited to.'*
- *'I take a long time to come, and when I do, it's like, 'Is that it?' My orgasms never seem as intense as other people's and I wonder if I'm doing something wrong – like maybe I'm missing something?'*
- *'Orgasming is a real challenge for me because penetration is painful, but my partner gets upset if I don't so I end up faking them all the time. I feel like I'm broken.'*

And it's not just them – in a survey of more than 1,000 American women, 59 per cent admitted to faking an orgasm.[4] Billie and I? Guilty as charged (on more than one occasion). What about you?

Then there's the infamous orgasm gap.[5] Our own survey of more than 11,600 people showed 81 per cent of men orgasm 'often to very often' during sex, while only 53 per cent of women said the same. An American study of over 52,000 adults echoes this, with a whopping 30 per cent difference between heterosexual men and women.[6] But here's the twist: in the same study, lesbian women orgasmed 86 per cent of the time. Likewise, in the *Hite Report*, a landmark study of women's sexuality, women orgasmed 92–95 per cent of the time during solo play.[7]

So, it's not about the female orgasm being 'more difficult' or women being 'less likely to come' – there's something else going on. In her book *Becoming Cliterate*, psychologist Dr Laurie Mintz explains that the orgasm gap is socio-cultural and not based on our biology.

But what if we shifted our focus from chasing orgasms to prioritizing pleasure?

How would sex be different? And how would we be different?

This chapter is all about exploring just that. We'll look at eroticism, the sensual side of sex, and how tools like mindfulness and savouring can enhance feelings of aliveness and your experience of pleasure. We'll also explore fantasies and your erotic imagination. By the end of this chapter, you'll have the tools to explore eroticism in your everyday life, tune into sexual sensations in your body, and prioritize your pleasure and erotic self.

Pleasure case study

Alright, let's break it down: as you might have gleaned by now, what goes on between the sheets and what happens in the rest of your life are more connected than Chandler and Monica in *Friends*. Life is chaotic and messy; we can't compartmentalize all the different parts into neatly organized drawers and expect it to stay that way. Pleasure is a prime example. That's because pleasure is about as personal as it gets – it's connected to our sense of self and what we're going through in our daily lives.

To shed some light on what it's like when the messiness of life gets in the way and your erotic self takes a back seat, let's hear a story from Billie.

PRINCIPLE 7 – PRIORITIZE YOUR PLEASURE

Billie's story

I kissed someone, and it wasn't Seb. I felt terrible, ashamed and pathetic. But, at the same time, there was a thrill, a sort of sense of aliveness and pleasure that I hadn't felt in a long time.

But I'm getting ahead of myself. Here's how it started . . .

After three years of waiting, Seb and I had finally carried out our plan to move to LA, but I'd been struggling to get my bearings, and in the transition I'd lost my sense of pleasure and aliveness. I was burnt out, missing my old routines and lacking community. I'd left a vibrant life in London and was trying to figure out how to create that for myself in a new place, but it wasn't going so well. Since moving, my mental health had been in a steady decline.

Yes, I was burnt out, but it was more than that. I recognized the familiar signs of depression – apathy, lethargy and a lack of interest in life – but I felt too numb and too low to do anything about it. I was incredibly isolated too. I had a wonderful community in the UK, and with the move I was a whole continent away from the people who energized and supported me. I felt disconnected from my erotic self, unable to access feelings of joy and aliveness or feelings of pleasure, both in sex and in life in general.

The realization of just how much I'd lost my sense of pleasure hit me when I went back to the UK for a retreat. During my visit, I felt the contrast between my two lives so sharply that it left me reeling. On the retreat, surrounded by my friends and other interesting and creative people, and engaging in activities that brought me joy, I felt that missing spark of life again. For the first time in a long time, I was buzzing, and I felt a sense of aliveness and pleasure. But with this newfound pleasure came a sense of dread.

I was only just beginning to shake off the numbness of the last nine months in LA. Everything in me screamed to hold on to anything I could and not let go.

It was on this retreat that I met Ryan. During a reflection activity, we had an honest and vulnerable conversation about where I was in my life and what I'd been feeling. He listened attentively, was curious and challenged me. I felt not only seen, but heard. The deeper we got, the more intriguing and alluring I found him. Our conversation further reignited a sense of aliveness inside of me — not just for life, but for sex.

After the retreat, Ryan and I ended up going out on a date.

I knew I shouldn't, but I was desperately trying to cling to the sense of aliveness I'd finally been able to access after months and months of dormancy. It was like I'd become intoxicated by this tiny bottle of joy that I'd found, and was drinking up as much as I could before it ran out. I was dreading going back to the US and I was terrified I'd lose my sense of pleasure again as soon as I got home.

It wasn't really about Ryan, but the escapism spending time with him provided. He was a form of avoidance — a distraction from the monotony, apathy and loneliness I'd been feeling in LA. It was like he woke up a part of myself that I'd been struggling to access on my own. But that was the problem — I needed to figure out how to access this part of myself in the reality of my daily life, not just in the temporary fantasy of being a world away from it.

When I got back to LA, I was completely derailed and my head was spinning.

I didn't feel numb anymore, I felt miserable. I was acutely aware of how low, lost and lonely I was feeling. Along with that came a profound sense of sadness and grief. I resented living in LA and leaving my life in London behind. My loss of pleasure

PRINCIPLE 7 — PRIORITIZE YOUR PLEASURE

returned, and this time, instead of apathy, I felt anger. I was angry at myself for what had happened with Ryan. I was also angry at Seb because I felt like if it weren't for our relationship, I would have chosen to move back home. And I was angry with LA, well, just because.

After I got back from the UK and the retreat, Seb and I talked about what had happened with Ryan and about how low I'd been feeling. I shared how being away from LA and back with my community had allowed me to feel joy, aliveness and pleasure again for the first time since we'd moved. The conversation was heartbreaking — for me, for Seb and for the future we'd planned.

I was desperately unhappy and knew something needed to change, but I had no idea what that something was. I felt like my autonomy was being taken away from me. If I wanted to be with Seb, I felt like I had no choice but to stay in LA. But if I stayed in LA, I was worried I wouldn't be able to get my sense of pleasure back and I'd end up even more depressed than I'd been the last nine months.

The whole experience was a wake-up call. I realized I wasn't asserting my agency and had fallen back into old behaviours of letting others dictate my life. I wasn't taking control of my situation or responsibility for my decisions, and I had used Ryan to distract myself from the loneliness, sadness and numbness I'd been feeling. In my vulnerability with Ryan, I had mistaken my desire to be seen and understood for my desire for sexual connection. What I needed wasn't a lover or a new partner to find my sense of pleasure again, but a coach or a therapist.

I needed to explore my insecurities and fears to understand and reframe them. I needed to figure out how to trust myself and reconnect my head and my heart. I needed to rediscover my erotic self *and sense of aliveness from within. I needed to find a way to access pleasure, not only in sex but in my life as a whole.*

The science: What you need to know about prioritizing your pleasure

Now, we've said it explicitly – that pleasure is more than orgasm. Pleasure is 'enjoying', and you experience it by cultivating feelings of aliveness and joy. As you saw in Billie's story, without these feelings, it's easy to lose touch with what brings us pleasure across all areas of our lives.

That being said, we know that orgasms are something a lot of folks are interested in learning more about, so we're going to take a pleasure pit stop and get to know some orgasm basics. We'll also throw a big old caveat in at the end too.

An orgasm is that moment when all the built-up sexual tension – both in your body and your mind – suddenly releases with a bang (or, more accurately, with involuntary muscle contractions). It's when your arousal hits its peak, or what we like to call the 'climax'. Usually this moment comes with a wave of relaxation, satisfaction and pleasure. Generally speaking, orgasms can last between twelve and twenty seconds, and bring about physical changes like an increase in heart rate and body temperature, rapid breathing and flushed skin.[8] Plus, during an orgasm, thanks to endorphins our pain tolerance goes up, and we get a rush of that 'feel good'

PRINCIPLE 7 – PRIORITIZE YOUR PLEASURE

dopamine and the 'love hormone' oxytocin. Orgasms can vary a lot in how they feel and how long they last, so they're not going to feel the same every time or for every person. Think of them like snowflakes – no two orgasms are exactly alike.

Getting into the nitty-gritty of orgasms can be tricky in clinical settings, but research does suggest that our orgasms feel similar across genders. In her book, *The Case of the Female Orgasm*, Elisabeth Lloyd talks about how the female orgasm is like a male nipple – it's a fun leftover from our shared developmental pathway. Basically, in the same way that male nipples aren't crucial for reproduction, the female orgasm seems to be more about pleasure than an evolutionary must-have.

When it comes to hitting that big O, around 72 per cent of women need a little (or a lot) of clitoral stimulation.[9] So, it's a safe bet that the clitoris is kind of a big deal in the pleasure department. But get this – we didn't even know the full anatomy of the clitoris until 1998, when Dr Helen O'Connell, a urologist, did the first full autopsy of it.[10] That's right, we made it to outer space before we fully explored what's going on 'down there'.

Here's a fun fact: when developing in utero (aka while in the womb), the clitoris and the penis start off the same. After about eight weeks, the Y chromosome in a male embryo kicks into gear and begins producing its own hormones. This is when the penis will begin to differentiate. Since they come from the same starting point, the clitoris and the penis are what scientists call 'homologous organs' – or as Dr Emily Nagoski says in

Come As You Are, 'the same parts, just organized in different ways'.[11]

The clitoris is honestly an amazing organ. Say it louder for the people in the back! It's the only organ in the human body that's purely for pleasure. With a whopping 8,000 nerve endings, it's our most sensitive, and it's a lot bigger than what you see on the outside – about four inches bigger, to be exact.[12] That so-called little button you see is just the tip of the iceberg, known as the 'glans' of the clitoris. The rest is hidden inside the body, looking more like a wishbone than a pea.

To keep the glans safe, the clitoris has a hood, kind of like a 'tent', formed by the labia minora or inner lips. And those shared origins we talked about? The hood's male equivalent is the foreskin. When things get steamy the clitoris fills with blood, like an erection, and can swell by up to 300 per cent.[13]

The clitoris hasn't had it easy – far from it in fact. It's been said that Galen, one of the most famous doctors of the Roman Empire, called it a failed attempt at a penis, while Italian anatomist Andreas Vesalius wrote it off as 'useless'.[14] Then there was the medieval Christian Church's witch-hunting guide in 1486, which dubbed the clitoris the 'devil's teat' and the way the devil 'sucked out his victim's soul'.[15] And let's not forget Freud in 1905, who kicked off the myth of the vaginal orgasm by saying that clitoral orgasms were inferior and immature.[16] Anatomically, that's basically like telling men to orgasm without touching their penis and making them feel bad if they can't. Oh, and Dr Charles Mayo Goss decided to remove the clitoris from *Gray's Anatomy* in 1948 – the

PRINCIPLE 7 – PRIORITIZE YOUR PLEASURE

go-to medical textbook. Even today, at least 200 million girls and women have undergone female genital mutilation, having their external genitalia partially or totally removed for non-medical reasons.[17] Needless to say, our bodies and our right to pleasure have had – and continue to have – a pretty tough go. If you want to dive deeper into these topics, we've included some great books as bonus reads at the end of this chapter.

This, combined with our own personal experiences, is what made Billie and I decide to start Ferly in the first place. We'd only just met, and found ourselves quickly becoming comrades-in-arms as we championed all-things-pleasure over a fifteen-minute lunch break. The one word that summarized what we were feeling? Angry.

While orgasms can feel great, and while tackling the orgasm gap is important because it's a sign of a bigger issue, orgasms aren't the be-all and end-all of pleasure. Pleasure is so much more. If we come back to pleasure as 'enjoying', there are loads of ways to enjoy sex and orgasms are just one option. When we start fixating on orgasms, we narrow down sex to this one goal or result, like hitting the jackpot. That turns sex and all the fun sexy activities into a mission to 'get off', rather than savouring the 'getting' along the way – like scratching an itch. Plus, it puts a ton of pressure on something that might not happen. Anorgasmia, low libido, performance anxiety – as a society we're so focused on the mechanics of how to 'do' sex, and how to do it 'right', that we make it all about function. Unfortunately, as Esther Perel and Alice Miller argue, in making it about function, we also create the idea of 'dysfunction'; rather than exploring the art of sex, we end up reducing it to its mechanics.[18]

Savour the whole meal, not just the last bite

To help you think about pleasure as more than orgasm, here's an analogy Billie and I like to use . . .

Imagine you've won a fancy, four-course dinner at a famous restaurant and you're taking someone you enjoy spending time with. From the moment you arrive and walk into the restaurant, you are met with a sense of wonder – the space is amazing. From the lighting, to the colours, to the textures, to the decor – everything about it feels considered, and designed to make you feel good. Maybe it has a view of the ocean or vineyards or a city skyline – or maybe it has no view at all, maybe it's dark, and intimate and cosy.

The service is equally impressive. From when you enter to when you leave, there are so many subtle and seamless details that elevate your entire experience. As you slowly make your way through your meal, you savour it. Each course has its own ritual and ceremony. You take your time noticing the shapes and colours of the food, and all the different smells. As you eat, you're surprised by the many flavours and textures, and the sounds in your mouth as you chew every mouthful, from the appetizers to dessert. There's no single moment about the evening that stands out to you; you're entirely immersed in all of it, present in your experience. It feels good, really good – it feels pleasurable.

Now, imagine it's the next day and you're telling one

of your best friends about it. What if you were to define your entire evening – from start to finish, whether it was good or not, how satisfied you were, how connected you felt, how 'worth it' it was – based on the 12–20 seconds of your last bite of dessert?

That's it.

Feels pretty silly, right? Maybe even a bit disappointing, to focus on only that last mouthful, even if it may have been your favourite part.

Not only does it reduce, ignore and dismiss your whole experience, it also puts a heck of a lot of pressure on that one last bite. But that's what we do when we focus purely on orgasm as the be-all and end-all of sex. We diminish and undermine our sexual experience as a whole, and ironically we also make it less likely to have an orgasm. By putting your pleasure front and centre instead, you can access broader, deeper and more erotic experiences – ones that nourish your body, mind and heart.

Explore eroticism and feelings of aliveness in your everyday

If you're looking to prioritize your pleasure, exploring eroticism is a must. And no, eroticism isn't just about lighting candles and playing John Legend. For all you history buffs, the word 'eroticism' comes from Eros, the ancient Greek god of love and sexual desire. But Eros wasn't only about sexual energy – he was a fan of creative energy too, and using it to help us live the good life. This is where the original roots of eroticism come from and why Billie and I think of eroticism like this:

> **Eroticism is your golden ticket to
> feeling alive and connected.
> It's about connecting to yourself, to others,
> and to the world around you – it's how
> you give meaning to your experiences.**

Eroticism is what makes sex and all our life experiences meaningful.[19] At its core, eroticism is an experience. When we say something is 'deeply erotic', it means we're fully dialled into it, using all our senses – sight, smell, sound, taste and touch – to savour every moment and give our experiences meaning.

Anthony Giddens, in his book *The Transformation of Intimacy*, explains that eroticism is about nurturing feeling and expressing it through our bodily sensations.[20] On a basic level, we use our senses to take in information and survive (hello, autopilot). But on an erotic level, we use our senses to create deep and meaningful connections that we experience through a feeling of aliveness. Think of it as turning from a 'just surviving' to an 'alive and thriving' playlist on your life's soundtrack.

Audre Lorde, in her essay 'Uses of the Erotic: The Erotic as Power', talks about how the erotic, through power and knowledge, acts as a guide:

> The erotic is . . . an internal sense of satisfaction to which, once we have experienced it, we know we can aspire . . . We can then observe which of our various

PRINCIPLE 7 – PRIORITIZE YOUR PLEASURE

life endeavours bring us closest to that fullness . . . When I speak of the erotic, then, I speak of it as an assertion of the lifeforce of women.[21]

Experiencing an erotic moment is about feeling alive. Exploring eroticism isn't just about the oo-la-la moments that come from sex (although those are good too). It's more about tuning into what feels sensual. If the sexual is about the physical act of sex, the sensual is about our experience of it.

Think about the dinner vs dessert analogy. Sensuality is like the restaurant; it sets the stage for pleasure because it invites you to be present and immersed in your experience – like being aware of your heart rate during an intimate moment, or noticing the warmth of your partner's skin or the faint sound of their breath in your ear. Eroticism creates a space for you to explore and tune into how you feel during sex, not just how you do it.

But it's also about so much more than what's happening in the moment; it's about all the moments around those moments too. That's because eroticism stretches way beyond the act of sex; it enriches your sensual experiences in your everyday life too. In *The Erotic Mind*, Dr Jack Morin writes, 'the erotic landscape is vastly larger, richer, and more intricate than the physiology of sex or any repertoire of sexual techniques . . . to make sense of it we must cultivate a whole new way of perceiving'.[22]

Imagine waking up to the golden light of the morning sun, hearing birds singing outside, smelling coffee brewing in the kitchen, taking that first bite of a fresh flaky croissant and feeling warm water sliding down your skin as you shower to start your day. Engaging our senses not only connects us more deeply to the world, but also to our erotic selves and our potential for pleasure in all the activities we do.

Eroticism and this sense of connection also helps us build our interoceptive awareness – fancy term alert – which is our ability to perceive and tune into our own body's sensations, like heartbeat, breath, muscle tension and arousal.[23] In the bedroom, eroticism and interoceptive awareness allow us to fully connect to our bodies, savouring sensations and connecting more deeply with all the potential ways we can experience pleasure.

When you start embracing these erotic moments in your everyday life, you're not only spicing up your sex life, you're also boosting your overall wellbeing and opening up a whole new world of opportunity for possibility, pleasure and being present.[24]

Bottom line: letting the erotic guide you isn't just about better sex; it's about living a richer and more vibrant life. So here's to living erotically – because who doesn't want to feel more alive, connected, and yes, a little bit sexy, every day?

The importance of being mindful

Try this real quick . . .

Take a deep breath in through your nose and slowly breathe out through your mouth. Repeat this three times.

PRINCIPLE 7 – PRIORITIZE YOUR PLEASURE

Focus on the sensations – the feeling of the rise and fall of your ribs and belly, the sight of any movement in your body, the sound of the air moving in and out, the taste in your mouth, any smells in the air . . .

If your mind wants to quickly race off, observe it and let it be.

Bring your attention back to your breath and the sensations in your body.

Well done! You just practised being mindful.

Thích Nhất Hạnh, a Buddhist monk and author of *The Miracle of Mindfulness*, describes mindfulness as 'keeping one's consciousness alive to the present reality'.[25] Putting it differently, Dr Jon Kabat-Zinn, a big name in making mindfulness mainstream, explains that mindfulness is 'the awareness that arises from paying attention, on purpose, in the present moment, and non-judgmentally'.[26] Whatever way you want to think of mindfulness, that's cool. The two main things you need to consider are: being aware of what's happening right now, and doing it with openness and acceptance.

It might feel like mindfulness is all the rage these days, but it's actually been around for about 4,000 years[27] – and for good reason. There's much evidence showing how mindfulness can help with everything from chronic pain and anxiety to boosting sexual function, desire and, yes, even orgasms.[28]

One of the main reasons for this is because it can help build your interoceptive awareness – a biggie for enjoying sex.[29] For example, women who went through an eight-session mindfulness programme reported a 60 per cent increase in desire, a 26 per cent boost in overall sexual function and a 20 per cent drop in sex-related stress.[30] Mindfulness also helps us savour the good stuff in life, which is key to amplifying the intensity and duration of how we experience pleasure.[31]

Contrary to what some might think, mindfulness isn't emptying your mind or floating away into some wonderfully blissful altered state – although you might. Instead, it's about paying close attention to whatever's happening right now, whether it's good, bad or meh, and letting thoughts, feelings and sensations happen, without trying to change or ignore them. Despite its name, mindfulness is less about being in your mind and more about being in your body. And that's where the erotic comes in. Mindfulness is itself erotic. It draws on your senses to connect you to those good old feelings of aliveness and pleasure.

While mindfulness and meditation are often lumped together, they're not quite the same. Meditation is a broader term for ritualistic practices that train the mind and bring about a certain state of consciousness. Mindfulness is more like a state of being, where you bring a quality of attention and presence to your everyday life. You don't need any special postures or mantras for mindfulness – you can do it anytime and anywhere, whether you're eating, walking or, yes you guessed it, having sex. To help get your mindfulness muscles moving, we've put together a fun and erotic tool for you later in the chapter, so stay tuned.

PRINCIPLE 7 – PRIORITIZE YOUR PLEASURE

Lean into your fantasies to unlock your pleasure

When you sleep, do you dream?

Trick question, everybody does. We might not always remember our dreams, but each and every one of us has them.[32] Sometimes our dreams make sense, but most of the time they don't. They can be strange and wondrous, often surreal, and sometimes plain kooky. So, here's the next question: have you ever woken up and thought to yourself or said to someone, 'I just had the weirdest dream'?

Generally, we don't feel all that uncomfortable talking about our dreams. In fact, the weirder they are, the more we feel the need to share them. And yet, when it comes to our fantasies, we close up faster than a clam at low tide.

Since starting Ferly, Billie and I have spoken to a lot of women about pleasure and one of the areas in which we can freely explore it most: fantasies. A surprising number have told us that, just as pleasure makes them feel indulgent or guilty, their fantasies do too, if they even give themselves permission to fantasize at all.

To the latter point – when we ask them if they daydream, they always say yes. Like with dreaming, we all daydream. At some point or other during our waking hours, our minds will inevitably wander off to la-la land. That's just what they do, and we don't think much of it.

A fantasy is just a daydream turned erotic. In *Mating in Captivity*, Esther Perel writes:

Sexual fantasy includes any mental activity that generates desire and intensifies enthusiasm. These thoughts need not be graphic, or even well-defined. They're often inarticulate, more feelings than images, more sensuous than sexual ... memories, smells, sounds, words, specific times of the day, textures – all can be considered fantasy as long as they set in motion the arc of desire.[33]

Whereas mindfulness helps you to become more present in your experiences, fantasizing is a complementary tool that allows you to do the opposite: to unlock feelings of pleasure by leaning into your imagination and disappearing into an entire erotic world that exists just for you.

As for feeling guilty, or even ashamed, for fantasizing – don't. You wouldn't feel guilty for having a dream, would you? By definition, fantasies aren't real. Just because you find yourself imagining someone or something, it doesn't mean you want it to happen in real life.

Here are some numbers to put your (erotic) daydreams at ease.

In his book *Tell Me What You Want*, Dr Justin Lehmiller shares how just normal fantasies can be. In a survey of 4,000 Americans, 80 per cent of people said they fantasized about having sex with multiple partners and 65 per cent fantasized about BDSM. Sixty-two per cent of women fantasized about being in an open relationship and 59 per cent of straight women fantasized about having sex with other women.[34] The takeaway? Fantasies come in all shapes and sizes, and among them

PRINCIPLE 7 – PRIORITIZE YOUR PLEASURE

there are some storylines that are a lot less taboo than you might think.

Think of fantasies as a sort of 'mental staycation' centred entirely around your pleasure. You can become whoever you want, wherever you want, and do whatever you want with whoever you want. Your fantasies might be romantic, adventurous or taboo. They might be about power and control, exhibitionism and voyeurism, or about having different partners or being different genders.[35] In your erotic mind, your fantasies can range from debauchery to delight.[36]

Your brain is one of the greatest sexual partners you could ask for, and it's dedicated entirely to pleasing you.

Fantasies aren't just for fun; they also serve several important roles in bringing more pleasure into our sex lives. Sure, they can turn us on and get us in the mood, but they do more than that. They're like a private pleasure playground where we can discover the depth of our sexuality and our eroticism without being bound by the real world or its constraints and consequences. By letting our imagination simply play, we can explore the boundaries of our sexual experiences and unlock new sides of our erotic selves.

For example, if someone's craving novelty or experiencing restlessness in their routine or responsibilities, they may fantasize about having sex with a stranger or strangers. If they're always having to be 'on' or 'in charge', they may fantasize about being more submissive and letting go of control. Fantasizing about threesomes or group sex may reveal wanting to be seen as a whole person, have your needs met or feel desired. And more romantic fantasies in secluded locations may relate to a desire for intimacy and connection alongside wanting to step away from life's distractions. While fantasies aren't necessarily literal, they can be a great tool to help us discover our intimate needs and how we might want pleasure to manifest in real life.

Dreaming is to fantasizing what sleeping is to having sex.[37] Our imaginations allow us to escape to other worlds and explore alternative dimensions, ripe with pleasure. Through our fantasies, we also tap into our erotic guide, which allows for both personal and profound discovery – as so aptly described by Audre Lorde. Our fantasies are windows into the self, and tools for self-discovery and personal growth. They're not random or meaningless, but instead reflect our subconscious desires and needs.

By understanding, integrating and even confronting our fantasies, we can address our underlying fears, insecurities and traumas, many of which block us from experiencing pleasure.[38] This empowers us to let go of shame, have greater self-acceptance and cultivate a more fulfilling and authentic sexual identity, which opens us up to feelings of joy and aliveness. Fantasies also allow us to connect our minds and bodies, which can help with arousal concordance – for instance, guiding your mind to be more focused on the sexual rather than distracted, allowing for more pleasurable experiences overall.[39]

PRINCIPLE 7 — PRIORITIZE YOUR PLEASURE

Prioritizing your pleasure in real life

There's nothing more personal than pleasure. Equally, there are few things that can feel more complicated. What turns you on one day can turn you off the next. That's why it's so important to know your mind, explore your body and build a practice of connecting the two. By accessing your erotic guide, you give words to the shape of your pleasure and acknowledge that it's a strange, wondrous and ever-changing thing.

Here's how Billie prioritized pleasure in her own life and found her way back to an even richer relationship with Seb and a joyful life in LA . . .

Back in LA, after what happened with Ryan and the heart-wrenching conversations with Seb, I knew that if I wanted to start experiencing pleasure in my daily life again, I had to prioritize it. I had to navigate through what was blocking me, find meaning again, and make my way back to my erotic self to not only enjoy sex, but also the richness of the world around me.

At the time, instead of daydreams and fantasies, I had nightmares. I imagined myself lost in a dense, dark forest, unable to find my way out. These were the realities I needed to confront and the tough decisions I needed to make. On the other side was a clearing, a life that felt pleasurable and truly mine. I knew the journey through the forest would be challenging, but I also knew I couldn't stay where I was any longer.

In losing my erotic self, I lost the guiding force in my life. Instead of being connected to myself and the world around me, my head and heart separated, and I became an observer, watching them battle it out as my life ticked by. This mind–body disconnect left me disoriented and lost – without that inner guide, I no longer trusted myself. I knew I had to get it back.

I decided to go on a five-day silent retreat.

It was rural and rustic, kind of like a camping trip but where you don't say anything to anyone the whole time. Every morning, I'd be woken up by a bell at 6 a.m. and eat breakfast, after which I'd spend the day meditating, sometimes in a group but most of the time alone.

The first day was hell.

Naively, I thought it would be a reprieve of sorts, something to protect me from the constant barrage of thoughts, insecurities and fears I was up against. It wasn't. If anything, being forced into stillness meant there was no way of running from them anymore. I was frustrated and angry. By the end of the day, I impatiently wrote in my journal that this was a mistake and I didn't get the whole meditation thing.

I also felt a sort of dopamine withdrawal. I'd spent the last year chasing pleasure and getting quick fixes from all sorts of places. Chocolate, Instagram, Netflix, porn, kissing Ryan. Sure, they felt good in the moment, but the feelings of pleasure didn't last long and would ultimately leave me feeling lower than before.

The second day was better.

Rather than trying to silence all the noise in my head, I told myself that I had six hours of meditating ahead of me, so I might as well accept it and get on with it already. This freed up space for me to pay attention to my senses – and if I'm being honest, there wasn't much else to do. I found a pond to sit by, and that's what I did: I sat. By the end of the day, I was in pain, all my muscles ached, and my back was stiff as hell, but I also felt the beginnings of calmness and a sense of being grounded. I was finally returning to my body.

PRINCIPLE 7 – PRIORITIZE YOUR PLEASURE

Day three was when my senses properly started to wake up. Suddenly, they went from a year of numbness to feeling very much alive. For the first time since starting to sit by the pond, I noticed turtles and frogs in it. Looking around me, I took in the vivid green of the trees and the gorgeous scent of blossoming flowers. I felt the warmth of the sun against my face and heard the wind whispering through the leaves. Eventually, as I sat still and repeated the mantra my teacher had given me out loud – 'Who am I, I am' – I went into a trance-like state. Pleasure started to flood not only through my body, but out of my body. I experienced it as this deep sense of groundedness and gratitude – this connection to myself and to everything around me. Like I was part of the world rather than just existing in it. It honestly felt like I was high. I was overwhelmed by so many feelings of aliveness that, to this day, it was one of the most fulfilling and joyful experiences I've ever had. I'd tapped back into my erotic guide and it was leading me towards my own internal sense of completion, fullness and pleasure.

The fourth and fifth days were much the same. I continued to savour the eroticism of every waking moment. From the warmth of the morning sun on my skin, to the sounds of the birds and the complexity of their songs, to the spices and rich flavours in my food, to the weight of my body anchoring itself to the ground beneath me, I felt present, connected and alive.

When I left, I left with the understanding that all the pleasure I needed was living inside of myself already. The challenge wasn't to get it back, it was to cultivate the space it needed to grow. Instead of savouring, I'd been numbing, and instead of fuelling myself with all the things that brought me pleasure, I'd been filling my life with short-term stimulants and distractions. The dense forest from my nightmare wasn't all these big life decisions – it was fear, shame and self-criticism.

I know that it might not be possible for you to take off for five days whenever you're feeling disconnected, but it is possible to close your eyes, tune into your senses and take a moment for yourself. That's the beauty of meditation and mindfulness – you can do them anywhere and apply them to anything. While I didn't practise meditation prior to that retreat and, not going to lie, I've only half kept it up, I do continue to practise mindfulness in my day-to-day life. From little moments like noticing the feeling of the water trickle down me as I take a shower or stopping to take in the flavours and sensations when I eat, to bigger moments like when I'm masturbating or having sex, tuning into my erotic self empowers me to connect my head and heart so that I feel present and aligned in my mind and body.

I often come back to a quote by Rumi that our teacher shared with us on that retreat: 'Close your eyes, fall in love, stay there.' Prioritizing pleasure means not only focusing on the pleasure you get from others but on the pleasure you give yourself. The most powerful place we can be is somewhere we can experience our aliveness from within. It's not just about knowing how to turn yourself on in the bedroom, but about feeling alive and connected to how we're feeling in every aspect of our lives. If you can do this, if you can embrace your pleasure with open arms and an open heart, your erotic guide can help lead the way to a more connected, fulfilled and joyful you.

Living a pleasurable life in the bedroom means living a pleasurable life outside of it too. Pleasure isn't having an orgasm, it's this huge, erotic landscape that goes way beyond experiencing sudden and involuntary muscle contractions. It's about being present, connecting and feeling alive in whatever we're experiencing, whether it's sexual or not. Pleasure is savouring the journey, not

PRINCIPLE 7 – PRIORITIZE YOUR PLEASURE

rushing to the finish line. By being mindful, tapping into our senses and exploring our fantasies, we empower our erotic selves to lead the way. When we make pleasure a priority in all aspects of our lives, we create a richer, more satisfying existence in everything that we do.

In practice: Here's how to prioritize your pleasure

Tool #1: Craft an erotic fantasy

Everyone fantasizes in some way, and this tool lets you tap into your erotic imagination through creativity and introspection. Exploring your erotic fantasies can be empowering, especially if it's new to you. Remember, fantasies are a normal and healthy part of your sexuality, and there's nothing wrong with a bit of erotic daydreaming.

For this exercise you'll need somewhere to write things down. If you'd like a bit of extra privacy, one option is to make a note in your phone and lock it so only you have access to it.

STEP 1: BRAINSTORM YOUR CONTEXT

- If you need to, give yourself permission to fantasize, knowing that fantasies aren't real.
- Think about what arouses and excites you, whether it's a feeling, image or memory, and note your body's response.

- Imagine a scene that engages all five senses: sight, sound, smell, taste and touch. The richer the sensory details, the more vivid your fantasy.
- Consider the emotional atmosphere you're curious about, such as passion, tenderness, adventure, romance or kink.
- Who is in your fantasy? It could be yourself, a partner, someone you know or an imagined figure.
- What dynamics play out between the characters? Think about power dynamics, emotional connections and interactions that excite you.

STEP 2: CREATE YOUR FANTASY

- **Begin your story:** Start with a setting that sets the tone for your fantasy.
- **Middle:** Develop the action. What is happening? This might involve a sexual act, seduction or an unfolding scenario.
- **Climax:** Build towards a climax, which might be a physical act, a revelation or a powerful emotional connection.
- **Resolution:** Conclude with a resolution. How does your fantasy end, and what emotions or state of mind does it leave you with?

PRINCIPLE 7 — PRIORITIZE YOUR PLEASURE

STEP 3: DO SOME AFTERCARE

- After writing your fantasy, reflect on your feelings. How do you feel? Excited? Curious? Nervous? Acknowledge these feelings as part of your erotic self.
- Reread your fantasy and make any adjustments to enhance the experience. This is your private creation, shaped by your desires.
- If comfortable, consider sharing your fantasy with a partner – or even better, have them write their own and share them with each other! If sharing a sexual fantasy feels like too much, opt to share a fantasy about things that bring you a sense of aliveness instead. This might look like talking about activities that bring you joy or physical places that make you feel grounded and connected.

Tool #2: Try an arousal awareness meditation

Get ready for a fun little erotic adventure you can do from the privacy and comfort of home. This tool helps you tune into your senses and become more aware of how different sensations feel in your body. Don't forget to set up your environment in a way that feels good before starting.

What you'll need:

- A private, comfortable space without interruptions

- A fantasy or some erotica (short story, illustration, graphic novel, ethical porn, etc.)*
- Optional: Lube and a sex toy of your choice (e.g. a vibrator)

As a heads-up . . . if using erotica or a sex toy makes you uncomfortable, of course go ahead without. But it would also be worth exploring where this discomfort comes from. For example, we've noticed a lot of women, particularly if they come from more conservative or traditional backgrounds, might feel embarrassment, judgement or even shame when it comes to their own pleasure. If you do, remind yourself that you're in the process of letting go of disempowering beliefs and your pleasure is your right.

Likewise, some women are choosing to take a break from things like porn and sex toys to slow down their sex lives and to disconnect from technology in their self-pleasure practice. Whatever you choose is up to you.

It's also okay to take time to work up to this practice. Remember, growth can come from stepping outside your comfort zone, and you can always stop at any time.

---

* Ethical porn is like a breath of fresh air compared to mainstream mass-market porn. It focuses on real consent, diversity and pleasure equality, avoiding the unrealistic and often harmful depictions you see in typical porn. Its production also values things like fair pay, health and safety, and protection for workers. For women looking to spice up their sex lives, ethical porn can be a great tool. It shows authentic ways people can enjoy intimacy, which can be both erotic and educational. Watching porn can be fun and a great way to increase desire, but it can also be good to take breaks from it too. Feel free to slow down, do a dopamine detox and tune into your own imagination when the mood takes you.

PRINCIPLE 7 – PRIORITIZE YOUR PLEASURE

Here are your step-by-step instructions:

1. **Set up your environment:** Create a mood that feels like going on a date with yourself. Dim the lights, light a candle, play some music and lock the door if possible. Keep your erotic stimuli and props close by.
2. **Get comfortable:** Lie down or sit comfortably with pillows to support your body. Relax and take deep breaths to settle in.
3. **Do a body scan:** Do a quick scan of your body from head to toe, noting any sensations or tight spots.
4. **Engage with props:** Spend 5–10 minutes engaging with your props. Immerse yourself in your fantasy or erotica, using your imagination to activate your senses. If using a toy, explore different parts of your body without aiming for orgasm.
5. **Return to your body:** Put your props aside and do another quick body scan. Notice any changes in your breath, heart rate, temperature or sensations. If there aren't any, that's okay too.
6. **Focus on your genitals:** Pay attention to any external and internal sensations in your genitals. Observe how you feel, without judgement. See if you can isolate different parts of your body and observe any changes or shifts in sensation. What, if anything, do you feel? Are these feelings good, bad, neutral? Do you want more of something or less of something?

7. **Practise mindfulness:** If your mind wanders, gently bring your focus back to your breath and your body. Take a few deep breaths.
8. **Reflect:** Spend a few moments in stillness, reflecting on your experience. Acknowledge any emotions – good, bad or in between – and thank yourself for this self-exploration.
9. **Journal:** Jot down any thoughts or feelings you have, or do a quick journal entry, so you can keep track and look back on changes in your experiences over time.

Tool #3: Stop masturbating, start self-pleasuring

This tool draws on the art of mindful masturbation, or self-pleasure. While masturbation often focuses on the physical act and the end goal of orgasm, self-pleasure encompasses a broader, more erotic approach. Self-pleasure is a form of self-care. It's about tuning into your body, savouring each sensation and embracing the experience without any pressure to reach a climax. It encourages you to slow down and explore your erotic self in a kind and present way. Remember that your body goes through changes, and so how you experience your body might change too. We've written the instructions below for vulva bodies; feel free to adapt them to whatever genitals you may have.

PRINCIPLE 7 — PRIORITIZE YOUR PLEASURE

Here are your step-by-step instructions:

1. **Create a comfy space:** As always, pick a spot where you won't be disturbed and where you can relax. Set the mood with some cosy lighting or candles, put some tunes or white noise on, and use pillows if you like. Grab any goodies you might want, like lube, towels or toys, and dress or undress in whatever way feels good for you. Set a timer for a minimum of fifteen minutes.
2. **Start with some deep breaths:** Close your eyes if you can and take a few deep breaths, breathing in slowly through your nose and out gently through your mouth. Focus on your ribs and belly moving up and down.
3. **Scan your body:** From the tips of your toes to the top of your head, slowly work your way up your body, noticing any spots that feel tight or relaxed. Let yourself feel whatever's there without judging it.
4. **Wake up your senses:** What can you feel, hear, smell and taste?
5. **Experiment with touch:** Start by lightly running your hands over your arms, legs and torso. Let your hands wander freely, with no goal in mind. Gently massage your chest and nipples, your hips and your thighs – take note of how it all feels. Play with pressure, pace and type of touch. Think about hard/soft, slow/fast, and tickling, tracing, massaging, pinching, tapping, etc.

6. **Discover down under:** With your fingers (and lube if you prefer), explore all the different parts of your vulva like your outer and inner labia, your clitoral hood and the entrance to your vagina. Experiment with touching your clit and notice what, if anything, feels good. Try out various pressures, paces and types of touch.
7. **Explore inside your body** (if you're up for it): If you're feeling it, gently slide a finger or two inside your vagina. Notice how different parts feel to touch. Experiment with making a 'come here' motion, swirling around or thrusting. Now, combine internal and external touch.
8. **Stay in the now:** Keep your focus on the sensations you're feeling. If your mind starts to wander, gently nudge it back to the here and now, and what feels good or what you're open to exploring. Link your breath with your movements, breathing in deeply as you touch and breathing out slowly as you let go and stroke. If you feel comfortable, experiment with making sounds – this can help you to let go.
9. **Take it slow:** If you start to get more turned on, you might want to up the ante with your touch. Follow what feels good. This isn't about rushing, it's about savouring. You could try edging – getting close to climax, then easing off to keep building arousal.
10. **Keep exploring:** Continue to play with touch until your timer goes off. If you want to go

PRINCIPLE 7 – PRIORITIZE YOUR PLEASURE

longer, feel free. Don't stress about having an orgasm. If it comes, ride it out. If not, great! You're practising self-pleasure rather than chasing a result.

11. **Do aftercare:** After you're done, take a moment to relax and soak in the sensations in your body. Think about what you experienced, and any thoughts or discoveries that may have popped up during your practice.

QUICK TIP

Use this visual guide that we've created to experiment with different types of clitoral play. Each image represents a different way of exploring clitoral sensations. This can be in your practice, or you can share it with a partner and sample each one as they make their way through the list.

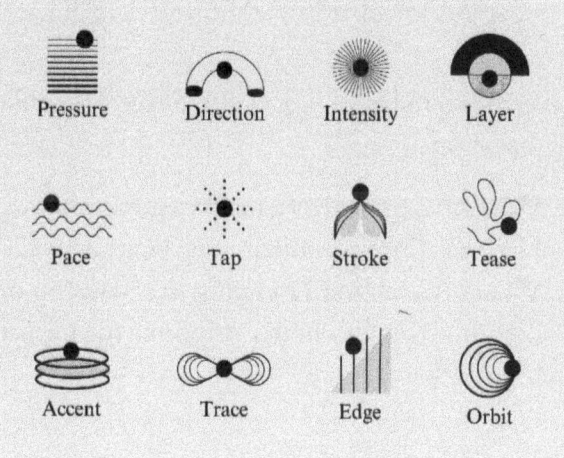

Pressure	Direction	Intensity	Layer
Pace	Tap	Stroke	Tease
Accent	Trace	Edge	Orbit

Tool #4 (surprise!): *10 minutes of play*

We thought we'd throw in a surprise partnered exercise for you to try out too. This one's simple.

Set a timer for ten minutes. One partner will give touch, while the other one does nothing but receive it. After ten minutes, switch.

Discuss the following ahead of time:

- Any areas you don't want touched or only want touched in a certain way.
- Whether or not you'd like to include genital touch, and if so, what kind. For example, clit play but no penetration.
- Have a 'no sex' rule. Agree to stop when the timer stops (even if you're aroused and want more – use that 'wanting' to build erotic tension rather than feeding it right away).

Look back to look forward

Take 1–2 minutes to reflect and answer the following questions:

1. How am I prioritizing my pleasure well?
2. How am I not prioritizing my pleasure well?
3. What's one action I'm going to start, stop or continue NOW to better prioritize my pleasure in my life?

PRINCIPLE 7 – PRIORITIZE YOUR PLEASURE

> If you'd like to dive deeper, we've hooked you up with some great resources and downloadable templates at www.turnyourselfon.co.

Cement your learnings

- Pleasure is not synonymous with orgasm. Pleasure is 'enjoying' whereas orgasm is a release of tension through sudden and involuntary muscle contractions.
- Having an orgasm is one of many ways to experience pleasure – remember to enjoy the whole experience of dinner, not just the last bite of dessert.
- Eroticism is about feelings of aliveness and connection. It's how you give meaning to your experiences both in and out of the bedroom.
- Each of us has an erotic guide that we access through our senses and by following our feelings of aliveness. Following your erotic guide can lead you to living a life of pleasure.
- Practices like mindfulness help you to connect mind and body so that you can build your interoceptive awareness and feel present in your experiences, and do so in a way that is open and accepting.
- We all have fantasies. Sometimes they're elaborative narratives, other times they're not. A fantasy is anything that adds to your pleasure

and creates a feeling of sexual 'wanting'. Fantasies are fantasies because they're not real. They're a tool you can use to help you discover your erotic mind, and learn more about your desires and what brings you pleasure.

Bonus reads

SOCIAL COMMENTARY

- Dr Laurie Mintz, *Becoming Cliterate: Why Orgasm Equality Matters – And How to Get It*
- adrienne maree brown, *Pleasure Activism: The Politics of Feeling Good*
- Nan Wise, PhD, *Why Good Sex Matters: Understanding the Neuroscience of Pleasure for a Smarter, Happier, and More Purpose-Filled Life*
- Anna Lembke, MD, *Dopamine Nation: Finding Balance in the Age of Indulgence*

SOLO EXPLORATION

- Debby Herbenick, PhD, *Because It Feels Good: A Woman's Guide to Sexual Pleasure and Satisfaction*
- Holly Richmond, PhD, *Reclaiming Pleasure: A Sex Positive Guide for Moving Past Sexual Trauma and Living a Passionate Life*
- Betty Dodson, PhD, *Sex for One: The Joy of Self-Loving*

PRINCIPLE 7 — PRIORITIZE YOUR PLEASURE

- Ev'Yan Whitney, *Sensual Self: Prompts and Practices for Getting in Touch with Your Body: A Guided Journal*
- Rachel E. Gross, *Vagina Obscura: An Anatomical Voyage*
- OMGYES, https://omgyes.com

PARTNERED EXPLORATION

- Emily Nagoski, PhD, *Come Together: The Science (and Art!) of Creating Lasting Sexual Connections*
- Meg-John Barker and Justin Hancock, *Enjoy Sex (How, When and If You Want To): A Practical and Inclusive Guide*
- Peggy J. Kleinplatz, PhD, and A. Dana Ménard, PhD, *Magnificent Sex: Lessons from Extraordinary Lovers*

FANTASY

- Online erotic stories: https://literotica.com; https://frolicme.com
- Erotic audio: Ferly App, Dipsea and Quinn
- Ethical and artful porn: https://erikalust.com

Principle 8 – Improve Your Communication

By reframing difficult conversations, navigating feedback and practising relationship repair

Real quick, here's a question for you: how confident do you feel talking to your partner about sex and asking for what you want in bed?

We asked nearly 12,000 people that question, and a whopping 71 per cent confessed they struggle to communicate confidently. That's right, about three-quarters of us are in the same boat, feeling like we're at a loss for words when it comes to talking about sex. It's pretty wild when you think about it – how can something like sex, which is so core to our human experience, be so tough to talk about?

Well, there's this outdated notion that sex is still taboo. Toss in some old-school gender norms and societal expectations telling women not to impose, make a fuss, be difficult, be bossy, be impolite – you get the gist – and you've got a recipe for communication chaos. Whether it's asking for what we want in bed, sharing how we feel or having a difficult conversation, the sad truth is a lot of us have never learned how to

PRINCIPLE 8 – IMPROVE YOUR COMMUNICATION

communicate effectively – if we were even encouraged to speak up at all.

And yet communication isn't a nice-to-have, it's a necessity. Research by relationship experts Dr John Gottman and Dr Julie Gottman shows that good communication is the number-one predictor of sexual and relationship satisfaction, and it's also the biggest determinant of whether a relationship will last. They also found that 69 per cent of conflicts in romantic relationships don't get resolved, and couples typically wait a staggering six years before seeking help.[1] It's no wonder so many of us feel like we're stuck in our heads. Rest assured if you find communication tricky, you're not alone – you're in pretty good company.

Here's what some women in our community had to say:

- *'I feel confident in pretty much every other part of my life, but when it comes to sex, I freeze. I don't know how to be sexy or relax in the moment or talk about what turns me on. I just wish I could communicate better.'*
- *'Every time we get intimate, my partner loses his erection. I don't know how to bring it up without making him feel worse. We just keep pretending everything's fine.'*
- *'I can orgasm by myself, but I've never been able to with my partner. We've been together for 12 years and I don't know how to approach it now. He is really loving, but he gets impatient when I try to give feedback, and rushes things. I can't stop thinking about how our sex might just be mediocre forever.'*

- *'Our fights can get pretty intense. I blow up, she shuts down. We both love each other so much, but our communication styles just clash. I want to learn how to express myself in the way that I want and not just see red.'*

It's clear that communication woes can throw a wrench in our love lives and overall sexual and relationship satisfaction. We get shares like these all the time from the women in our community. Communication sits at the heart of all our relationships, romantic and otherwise. And it's not only with the romantic stuff that our words fail us. At work, 89 per cent of us wrestle with ineffective communication, and a third of us regularly deal with co-worker conflicts.[2] Don't even get us started on the drama that can happen with friends and family. Navigating communication can feel like trying to solve a Rubik's cube blindfolded – damn near impossible. Yet it doesn't have to be.

From knowing your intimate needs to building your confidence, communication is a skill that builds on everything else you've learned so far. That's why we've saved the best (and trickiest) principle for last. If you can get the hang of talking about your deepest desires and expressing yourself in your most intimate and vulnerable context, talking about anything else in life gets much easier.

Whether you're the type to avoid confrontation, the one who's ready to debate at the drop of a hat, or somewhere in the middle, this chapter is your guide to levelling up your communication game. We're not going to

PRINCIPLE 8 – IMPROVE YOUR COMMUNICATION

sugarcoat it – becoming a master communicator doesn't happen overnight. It's a skill that needs practice and patience. By the end of this chapter, you won't be an expert (yet), but you'll be better equipped to have difficult conversations, navigate feedback and repair your relationships after a spat. Armed with the knowledge of what good communication looks like and the tools to practise it, you'll be all set to find your power and speak more confidently, both in the bedroom and beyond.

Communication case study

Nobody enjoys talking about hard things. Whether it's with partners, co-workers, friends or family, certain conversations can make us feel really nervous. From expressing our needs to handling feedback to navigating conflict – by definition, difficult conversations are, well, difficult. But they're also necessary.

To show you what not-so-great communication looks like and how it can impact our various relationships in real life, I've got a story to share. It's about how I not only failed to communicate well, but to communicate altogether.

Anna's story

With my back against the door, I sat down on the bathroom floor and tried to get control of myself. I had already turned the tap on – I didn't want him to know how upset I was and that I was crying. In between sniffling and wiping my nose, I tried to undo my lace corset but I kept fumbling with the clasps. My hands were shaking from all the feels. It'd taken me nearly fifteen minutes to put this stupid thing on. I'd barely worn it a minute before he covered his face with his hands, turned away from me and told me to change.

It was 2018 and Adam and I were still newish. We'd only been together for about half a year and we were already having problems. In the first three months, we hadn't been able to keep our hands off each other. As for the last three, we'd not had sex once and he'd been struggling to get hard. Unlike my five-year relationship with Tim, this time it was me with the higher desire. It wasn't just our lack of sex that was worrying me though, it was the lack of any touch at all. We barely hugged anymore and the only kisses he awarded me were quick pecks in passing when I did something nice.

His lack of physical affection left me feeling like I couldn't pleasure him, like I was unattractive and unwanted, and like I wasn't enough. The more disconnected we became, the more self-conscious I grew. With every kind rejection and gentle recoil, I felt more and more like a part of me was wrong and there wasn't space for it anymore. It was like I needed to seal my sexuality up in a box and quietly tuck it away somewhere, leaving it to be forgotten as life went on.

The weekend before, we'd gone away and he'd mentioned feeling connected afterwards. He was more physically affectionate too. He'd held my hand and played with my hair, pulling me close as we fell asleep together. I took it as an invitation to try again. I decided I would mix it up, do something different. My hope was that I could create an opportunity for us to get out of our heads, to go back to how we used to be, to rediscover one another anew. It seemed I'd misread the signals.

So here I was crying on the bathroom floor, angrily stuffing

PRINCIPLE 8 – IMPROVE YOUR COMMUNICATION

lingerie back into my bag. There was a lot of noise going on in my head.

Why does Adam get to dictate our sex life?
What about what I need?
Why is it always about him?

I felt angry and defensive. Then, I immediately felt guilty for feeling anything other than supportive. I understood what he was going through – that he was feeling confused, conflicted and ashamed. I'd been there myself with Tim, years before. I knew how debilitating and humiliating low desire and performance issues can be. Even though I was hurting, I told myself that Adam's hurt was more. It was neither empathetic nor fair of me to be upset. Along came more noise in my head.

What was I thinking, putting this kind of pressure on him?
How could I be so selfish?
I'm a horrible person.
Oh my god, I'm becoming Tim.

The thought of behaving like my ex made me feel physically ill. My anger redirected itself inwards. It found an easier target – myself.

I should be more supportive.
I should have more control over my feelings.
I should respect his needs more.
I shouldn't put pressure on us to have sex.

I was determined to be a better partner, to be a better person. I stood up and splashed my face with cold water. Taking a few deep breaths, I steadied myself against the sink.

Putting my pyjamas back on, I returned to the bedroom and slipped into bed next to him. He didn't move. He kept his back to me and said nothing. Trying to make things better, I reached out and wrapped my arms around his waist. 'I'm sorry,' I whispered as I curled up against his back. He didn't answer. My eyes welled up once more.

Calm down.

Stop making a big deal of everything.

You're fine.

As my silent tears wet the pillow, he finally drifted off to sleep.

I knew we needed to have a difficult conversation, but I couldn't bring myself to have it. Neither could he. And so we swept it under the rug and carried on like everything was fine, as if 'fine' was a thing to strive for. We trudged along, both of us unhappy and stuck in a sort of relationship limbo, each held hostage by our own inability to communicate and have the conversation we both so desperately needed.

And it wasn't just in the bedroom that I was struggling to communicate; the same pattern was slowly bleeding into other areas of my life too. The more things I had on, and the more responsibilities I was juggling, the more my inability to communicate kept getting in the way. While I struggled to articulate my needs the most with Adam, I was facing the same challenge in my other relationships. It resurfaced in people-pleasing with friends, leaving things unsaid with family and failing to set boundaries with work.

Both in and out of the bedroom, I struggled to communicate because I was afraid of hurting the other person's feelings or having mine hurt in return. More than that though, I struggled to communicate because I'd never learned what good communication looked like. It was never modelled for me, in the same way that it was never modelled for my parents, nor for theirs.

I think that's the case for most of us. We live in a world that

PRINCIPLE 8 — IMPROVE YOUR COMMUNICATION

tells us that communication is the most important skill we'll ever have, and yet no one has ever actually taught us how to do it.

Unfortunately, the world's right – about this at least.

Being good at communicating changes everything, just as being bad at communicating does too. The difference is that good communication makes things infinitely better whereas bad communication makes things infinitely worse.

That was my problem.

But how could I learn what good looked like when I'd so far had nothing to compare good to?

I didn't have difficult conversations because I didn't know how. I didn't do feedback well because I didn't know how. I didn't do relationship repair because I didn't know how (or that it was even a thing).

I knew communication was important, desperately so. I also knew it was expected of me and it was something I was supposed to be good at. Despite all that, my communication struggled. I had no idea what it meant to communicate well, let alone how to do it in practice.

The science: What you need to know about communication

We often think of 'communication' as talking about our feelings. Sure, that's a big part, but there's so much more to it. Let's geek out here for a minute. It'll help to make sense of all the layers of communication later.

So, starting from the top.

Communication is how we exchange information

so we can connect, share and understand each other. We do this through a mix of words and body language. In any interaction we have, there are two roles that we move back and forth between in conversation: the giver and the receiver. The switches happen quickly, continuously and sometimes even simultaneously. The giver sends the message (that's called 'encoding'). This could be words, but it could also be a smile, a scowl or a shrug. Then, the receiver interprets the message (that's called 'decoding'). Both roles are key because the way we send and receive a message allows us to know if we're on the same page.

Sounds simple, right?

Trick question. We all know it's not. While we might like to think of communication as a simple back-and-forth, it's rarely that easy. That's because communication is all about context. Whether it's the environment, the situation, how a message is sent or received, the relationship between the giver and receiver, or what the message is – there are loads of things that impact how clearly information is shared (or not).

The point here isn't to make communication seem even more intimidating, but to reassure you that there's a lot at play when we communicate, and some of it is out of our control. Be kind to yourself. Your aim isn't to get it right every time, but to instead get a bit better with each try.

Cool?

Cool. Now, the moment you've all been waiting for: how to have a difficult conversation.

PRINCIPLE 8 – IMPROVE YOUR COMMUNICATION

*How to have a difficult conversation:
See it as a threefold approach*

The reason that difficult conversations are more complex than an easy-breezy chat about the weather is because you're actually juggling three conversations all at once: the 'What Happened?' Conversation, the Feelings Conversation and the Identity Conversation. This little gem comes from Douglas Stone, Bruce Patton and Sheila Heen's book *Difficult Conversations: How to Discuss What Matters Most*. To help you communicate better, we're going to draw on some of their research to describe each of the three conversations.

THE 'WHAT HAPPENED?' CONVERSATION

The first conversation is about what we believed happened or should happen.

This one's about your perception of events, or where you interpret a sequence of events differently. For example, say you're late to your date. You think it's because of traffic, which was outside of your control and it's not a big deal – there was nothing you could do. Your partner, however, thinks you should have left earlier, and takes your tardiness as a signal that the evening isn't as much of a priority to you as it is to them.

The 'What Happened?' conversation is a bit of a time and energy drain, because it often goes in circles and gets easily derailed by disagreements. We tend to make three assumptions here: we're right, we know the other person's intentions, and they're to blame (and of course, we're not).[3] Also? Just as you're making assumptions, the other person is too.

Remember the whole 'thoughts aren't the same as facts' piece from chapter 3? Just because you assume something doesn't make it true.

For example, I had assumed it was okay for me to initiate (that I was right) because Adam had been more physically affectionate on our weekend away, and so I thought he was open to having sex again (thinking I knew his intentions). I also assumed it was Adam's fault for sending me mixed signals (that he was to blame).

From Adam's perspective, he might have assumed it was fine to reject my initiation, cover his face and tell me to change out of my lingerie (that he was right). He may have assumed he'd made it clear to me and that I knew he still wasn't interested in having sex with me (thinking he knew my intentions). He also may have faulted me for trying to initiate and putting him in an uncomfortable position where he felt he had to reject me (that I was to blame).

Looking back, instead of acting on my assumptions, I should have shared them with Adam and asked him for clarification to help me understand where I might have gotten things wrong. I also should have tried to remove my feelings from identifying 'what happened?' and instead been as objective about the facts of the situation as possible (more on this below).

PRINCIPLE 8 – IMPROVE YOUR COMMUNICATION

THE FEELINGS CONVERSATION

The second conversation is about how you feel, how others feel and whether those feelings are valid.

It may have been cool to brag about 'turning off' your feelings back in the day, but the reality is, you can't. It's not about whether your feelings will surface, but how to handle them when they do. Here's an example: you've had an argument with your partner and they want to talk about it, but you've shut down. You tell them, 'I'm fine,' and they tell you, 'You're obviously not fine.' Deep down you're feeling angry, stuck and unable to articulate how you feel. At the same time, they're feeling frustrated, resentful and like they're not allowed to articulate how they feel. Neither of you is having the Feelings Conversation, but both of you have feelings that are surfacing and getting in the way.

According to Stone, Patton and Heen, unexpressed feelings can make your conversations difficult by leaking, bursting or blocking. You can see this in my situation with Adam. When they leak, they seep into your tone of voice, your facial expressions and your body language, like him covering his face and asking me to change. When they burst, they explode in actions like yelling, crying or storming out – take me sitting on his bathroom floor having a big old sob. Last, when feelings block, they get in the way of being able to listen, which limits how we receive messages and our ability to understand. You can see this in my own inner dialogue, where I blocked myself and my own feelings by prioritizing his, as well as when he rolled over and ignored my apology.

Had I known about the Feelings Conversation at the time, I would have shared the conversation I was having in my head about being angry and feeling guilty, instead of going round and round in circles on my own. I also would have told Adam how I felt when he pulled away from me, and that while I was happy to give him some time and space, there was a much bigger conversation we needed to have about how both of us were feeling about our sex life and our relationship as a whole.

THE IDENTITY CONVERSATION

The third conversation is the one you have with yourself about who you are as a person.
This is the trickiest conversation to untangle because it's introspective. It's what you tell yourself about yourself. Imagine you're in a relationship and your partner has shared they don't think you contribute to planning dates and prioritizing time together as much as they do. All those immediate thoughts that pop up like, 'Well, I do more around the house compared to them' and 'I feel guilty because of what they shared and so I must be a bad partner' – those make up the Identity Conversation.

Stone, Patton and Heen argue that when having a difficult conversation there are three main threats to our identities that get in the way of communicating successfully. These are doubts about our competence, goodness and worthiness of love.

Bringing it back to my experience with Adam, you can see how these three threats to my identity played

PRINCIPLE 8 – IMPROVE YOUR COMMUNICATION

out in real time with negative thoughts like: 'I'm bad at pleasing him, which is why he doesn't want to have sex with me' (competence); 'I'm a horrible person for creating this situation' (goodness); and 'I'm unwanted and not good enough' (worthiness of love).

Looking back, had I done the foundational work to build my own self-esteem when this happened, my Identity Conversation may have been a little less self-critical and a whole lot kinder to myself. For example, 'There are many reasons why Adam's libido might be low and it doesn't mean I'm bad in bed' (competence); 'I'm a caring and empathetic person who sometimes makes mistakes' (goodness); and 'I'm worthy and deserving of love' (worthiness of love). I also would have been better able to recognize my cognitive distortions ('should' statements, catastrophizing, minimizing, etc.) and to identify and reframe my disempowering beliefs (see chapter 3). This would have made it easier to put some distance between myself and the situation so that I could have more clearly and confidently had the difficult conversation both Adam and I needed.

Learn how to navigate feedback

Now that you know what goes into a difficult conversation, it's time to tackle how to actually have it. Remember when we mentioned science coming in handy?

This is why . . .

When it comes to improving your communication, particularly during difficult conversations like how to ask for what you want, you need to learn how to both give and receive feedback. To give you a real-life example of this gone wrong, I'm going to walk you through an argument I had with Luke. I'll start with what happened, explore three common triggers, and end with an overview of what went wrong and how Luke and I could have handled things differently.

Starting with how it all went down...

About a year ago, Luke and I were making dinner. From changing careers, to managing debt, to going to grad school, we had a lot going on. In between chopping garlic and sautéing onions, I mentioned to Luke that I wasn't sure what my next move with work should be, especially if we were thinking about having kids.

What started as an 'I wonder...' comment led to a conversation about money, which was followed by a discussion about job security, which ended in an argument about being a responsible parent. We both got defensive, which led to a back-and-forth of counterattacks. He rolled his eyes and walked out of the kitchen. Taking the pan off the stove, I followed him upstairs.

'Are you okay?' I asked Luke, as he sat down on the bed and started reading his book.

'Yeah. I'm fine.'

'You're obviously not fine. What's going on?' He didn't answer and instead kept reading. 'Do you want to talk about it?'

'No, not right now.'

'Okay. When do you think you'll want to talk about it?' I pushed.

'I don't know,' he immediately replied.

I audibly sighed and shook my head. 'You never know,' I mumbled.

PRINCIPLE 8 – IMPROVE YOUR COMMUNICATION

He rolled his eyes and continued to read. I kept staring at him, waiting expectantly for an answer.

'What?' he snapped.

'Nothing,' I snapped back.

'Okay.'

'Okay.' After a few minutes of silence, I walked across the bedroom and unplugged my phone charger.

'Where are you going?' he asked, putting his book down.

'To my parents'.'

'Now?'

'Yeah, it feels like you need a bit of space.' His expression was grim. 'I think it's better if I crash there for the night.'

'Okay, if that's what you want.' Turning away from me, he rolled onto his side and kept reading. I stood at the door waiting for a moment and then walked out the room.

Now that you know what happened, before I dive into our mistakes and how Luke and I could have done things differently, we're going to pause here for a second.

So far, we've learned that communicating well relies on having an awareness of the three conversations ('What Happened?', Feelings and Identity) as well as both giving and receiving feedback. There is, however, one more thing that can make communication tricky: triggers.

Triggers are the touchpoints that can cause us to have a strong emotional, psychological or physiological reaction. Say you're the type to avoid conflict, triggers can lead to defensive responses like shutting down, going silent or giving someone the cold shoulder. On the flip side, if you're more confrontational, triggers can make you 'see red', lash out or say things you don't mean.

To take a closer look, we're going to circle back to the communication wizards Douglas Stone and Sheila Heen. This time we're drawing on insights from another one of their books: *Thanks for the Feedback: The Science and Art of Receiving Feedback Well*. According to Stone and Heen, there are three sneaky triggers you need to watch out for.

WHY WE GET DEFENSIVE: THREE COMMON TRIGGERS

#1 Truth triggers: These happen when we think feedback is wrong

Sometimes the feedback we get isn't what we expected or what was intended. For example, Stone and Heen explain how we often mix up different types of feedback, like when someone gives us appreciation (saying 'thanks') versus coaching (saying 'here's a better way to do this') versus evaluation (saying 'this is where you stand').[4] Other times, we might get feedback we didn't ask for or don't know what to do with. These situations can lead us to doubt the accuracy, fairness or validity of feedback, and to dismiss it, get defensive or go on the offensive if we think it's 'untrue'.

For example, when I brought up the hypothetical about having kids in my conversation with Luke, I had intended for us to have a casual chat about it. Instead,

PRINCIPLE 8 – IMPROVE YOUR COMMUNICATION

it turned into me receiving unintended feedback in the form of an evaluation about my current job and how it didn't offer financial security or benefits whereas others might. While Luke wasn't trying to start a fight and was only trying to offer his perspective, I was caught off guard as I felt like I hadn't asked for feedback, and nor did I know what to do with the feedback he gave. This left me feeling under attack and like I needed to defend myself.

#2 Relationship triggers: These are about our relationship to the feedback giver and how we feel they treat us

Depending on our relationship with the feedback giver, we might not take their feedback so well. For instance, if we have a rocky relationship or we don't feel valued or respected by them, we're likely to ignore what they say. We get stuck on the 'who' behind the feedback instead of the 'what' of their words. We might even start to doubt their credibility, trustworthiness or motives. More real talk? A relationship goes two ways. You too play a role in shaping its dynamics.

In the context of the argument that Luke and I had, I dismissed some of Luke's feedback because I was receiving it from him rather than from someone who I perceived to be in a similar position to me. For example, had it been from a woman who had decided to have kids while also continuing to run her own business, I may have been more responsive and receptive. By dismissing Luke, I was closing myself off to his potential insights, creating tension in our relationship, as well as being condescending towards my partner and his own experiences.

#3 Identity triggers: These are tied to our sense of self

As we saw when exploring the three conversations, a lot of our ability to communicate well comes down to how we feel about our identities and whether we see ourselves as competent, good and worthy. We're prone to be triggered and to react poorly to feedback that challenges how we see ourselves and our world view.

During our argument, what Luke was trying to say was that, as a couple, we needed to think about financial security differently if we wanted to have kids. What I heard and internalized was that if I started another business instead of getting a 'proper job', I was being irresponsible and would be a bad parent, which threatened my sense of identity. It wasn't at all what Luke was communicating; it was my ego getting triggered as I made assumptions and jumped to the wrong conclusion.

Plus, as if communication isn't challenging enough as is, individual differences in our biology mean that how we perceive and experience feedback can vary by up to 3,000 per cent.[5] This makes identity triggers pretty personal. What sets you off and how you experience a situation might be different to how it affects someone else, or it may not even bother them at all. You can see some examples of how personal triggers can be in the different perspectives of how Luke and I experienced our argument . . .

PRINCIPLE 8 – IMPROVE YOUR COMMUNICATION

RECOGNIZING TRIGGERS:
LUKE AND ANNA'S DIFFERING
PERSPECTIVE ON OUR ARGUMENT

Now that you have an overview of how triggers can also impact our ability to communicate effectively and that they're incredibly personal, let's come back to what happened with Luke. When I asked him about it, this is what he shared:

Communicating with Anna can trigger me in two main ways. First, she wants to talk about things right away whereas I need time. I need time not only to work through what I'm feeling, but to figure out how to articulate it too.

The second trigger is how she quickly forms logical arguments about what's happened and moves on, while I'm still trying to process everything. This leaves me feeling incompetent and like I'm failing as a partner. I end up feeling stupid for not having a quick response, guilty for being a bad partner and ashamed of my behaviour.

It's like I'm stuck in this pit, beating myself up with self-criticism. I might look 'shut down', but my mind is racing. I'm replaying everything and ruminating on how I've hurt her and how she's hurt me, which feels even worse because we care about each other so much. What I want is to work through what I'm feeling, have a conversation, and reach out and help resolve things, but I can't seem to find my way out. This makes me even more angry at myself and feel even more incompetent as a person and partner, which starts the whole cycle over again.

Physical touch helps because it reminds me that I'm loved, but the timing has to be right. If it's too early, I push it away because

I'm still judging myself so harshly that I don't feel like I deserve it. What also helps is that Anna often gives me the benefit of the doubt and tries to understand what I'm feeling, which reassures me that I'm not a bad person.

On the flip side, I experienced our argument a lot differently. When I looked back on it and took some time to think about my own triggers and where they come from, this is what I discovered:

I get triggered when Luke stonewalls. I understand he's not trying to be difficult or doing it on purpose – he's genuinely overwhelmed and stuck in a sort of 'freeze' state. It's tough seeing him upset, and it's even harder knowing that I've played a part in it. It makes me feel like a bad person and like I need to fix things.

This stems from my own upbringing and being parentified as a child, where I was pushed into an adult role early on within my family. Growing up around a lot of erratic behaviour, I've become hyper-aware of how people are feeling. I often find myself monitoring their moods and anticipating changes in their behaviour as a way of feeling safe. If I notice something is off, I immediately feel like it's up to me to fix it, like I need to make things better and make sure everyone is okay.

This makes me default to a 'solving mode' during conflict. Unfortunately for Luke, when I do, I don't give him the time to work through what he's feeling. It's also a bit of a chicken-or-egg thing because his withdrawal triggers my need to fix, and the more I try to fix, the more he withdraws. This makes me pushy and domineering, and sometimes I also end up infantilizing him, which neither of us wants.

PRINCIPLE 8 – IMPROVE YOUR COMMUNICATION

What helps calm my triggers is reassurance. This might be Luke asking for space while also making sure to tell me he loves me, and once he's moved through his feelings, we can reconnect and chat through what's happened. I also find it helpful when he lets me know he's tired, hungry or stressed, and pauses a conversation before it escalates. This way, I don't misread his moods or feel like it's something I've done versus him not having capacity.

GIVING FEEDBACK WELL: SITUATION, BEHAVIOUR, IMPACT AND ACTION

Now that you understand the three different parts that make up difficult conversations, and how you or someone else might be triggered, you'll be in a much better place to communicate feedback and ask for what you want, in the bedroom or elsewhere. We hope you feel a little more equipped to navigate those conversations, whether it's telling a friend that you were upset when they didn't return your call, telling your boss that you're struggling with something at work or suggesting something new to try in the bedroom. Giving feedback isn't the same thing as criticizing someone, even though it might sometimes feel that way. Remember, criticism is an attack on someone's character or personality, and it never ends well for anyone.

A super-helpful guide for you to follow when giving feedback is the Situation, Behaviour, Impact and Action (SBIA) framework. First proposed by Sloan Weitzel and the Center for Creative Leadership, this framework is now widely used, and it's one that Billie and I both find really valuable in our professional and personal lives.[6] It's easy to follow and made up of four parts:*

1. **Situation: Set the scene.** This is a factual, objective statement about when and where the behaviour happened, giving some context for the feedback. Make sure you avoid using absolutisms (always, never, every time, etc.).
2. **Behaviour: Describe the specific actions that were observed.** This is a neutral and objective account of what the person did or said, without any assumptions about their intentions or character. It does not include judgement or blame.
3. **Impact: Describe the effects of the behaviour.** This is how the person's actions impacted the feedback giver and what the giver is thinking and feeling. It uses 'I' statements instead of 'you' statements.
4. **Action: Suggest a solution.** This is about what's going to be different moving **forward** or how you'd like the situation to change. It's also a great chance to practise setting boundaries (see p. 40).

---

* The original framework from the Center for Creative Leadership focused on the Situation, Behaviour and Impact elements. Over the last decade, it's been well received and adopted, with some of the newer iterations including the addition of the 'A' for Action.

PRINCIPLE 8 — IMPROVE YOUR COMMUNICATION

EXAMPLES OF HOW TO GIVE FEEDBACK WELL

If you want to up your communication game, this structure is a helpful one to follow. You might find the SBIA framework feels forced and formulaic at first, but that's okay. Trust us, it'll become more natural with practice. Here are some examples of how it can play out in real life:

With a partner...

'On Thursday night, I went to bed early because I was feeling tired and had an early morning (*situation*). When you got into bed later, you tried to initiate (*behaviour*). I felt guilty for not being in the mood and frustrated because I'd communicated that I was tired (*impact*). Next time, instead of watching Netflix after dinner, I'd love for us to go to bed earlier together so that we can have intimacy time without me being stressed about getting a good night's sleep (*action*).'

With a family member or friend...

'Remember last Saturday at brunch (*situation*)? I noticed you were on your phone and replying to emails (*behaviour*). It kind of bummed me out because I was looking forward to some quality time and catching up together without distractions (*impact*). Next time we grab a meal, how about we both keep our phones off the table so we can have a proper chat (*action*).'

With a colleague...

'After that two p.m. meeting today, when I got back to my desk, you popped over for a chat (*situation* and *behaviour*). Don't get me wrong, I love our catch-ups, but I felt distracted and under pressure because I had some tasks I needed to wrap up (*impact*). Next time, could we schedule a catch-up during lunch or after work (*action*)? That way, I can make sure I'm not swamped.'

> ### QUICK TIP
>
> This is a great tool to use to ask for what you want in bed or give your partner sexual feedback in a way that helps to avoid defensiveness.
>
> *Example:*
> 'The last few times we've had sex (*situation*), I noticed you climaxed first and we kind of finished after that (*behaviour*). I felt a bit disappointed because I hadn't quite finished yet and would have liked to keep going (*impact*). Next time, if one of us climaxes before the other, it would be nice to check in and see if the other wants to keep going (*action*).'

Your turn to give it a go...

Think back to a recent situation where you felt upset, frustrated or annoyed. Picture yourself giving someone feedback. How would you lay it out using the SBIA framework? Give it a shot, even if it's just in your head.

PRINCIPLE 8 – IMPROVE YOUR COMMUNICATION

Notice if it feels different from how you usually give feedback (if you do at all). Complete this little exercise and you'll have already levelled up your communication skills – big ups!

Connect after conflict: Relationship repair

When it comes to improving how we communicate, it's also important to think about what we do after. Disagreements, arguments and conflict are all a part of being in a relationship, whether that's with a partner, a friend or a colleague. Healthy conflict helps us grow and build stronger relationships through a process of rupture and repair. 'Rupture' is when something causes disconnection in a relationship, and 'repair' is when you acknowledge a rupture and start the process of reconnection.

Experiencing rupture feels like being out of sync and losing trust in your relationship – it's that 'ugh' moment. For example, when you have a fight with your partner or one of you fails to follow through on a commitment. Repair is your way of shaking off that 'ugh'. Since every relationship is unique, the way you mend things with your partner is going to be different from how you do it with a colleague or friend. The aim of repair is to rebuild trust and connection while also deepening your understanding of each other. Usually, this involves a conversation where you open up about your feelings, say sorry and offer forgiveness.

Keep in mind an apology doesn't sound like 'I'm sorry but . . .' because the word 'but' negates the apology by implying there's a justification or excuse for hurting someone else's feelings. Same goes for 'I'm sorry you feel that way', which implies the problem lies with the other person's feelings or reaction rather than taking responsibility for one's own wrongdoing. A proper apology – and one that can lead to repair – includes acknowledging the mistake, expressing genuine remorse and taking responsibility for an action and its impact on others.

Also, if you're going to forgive someone, you've got to let go of any resentment, grudges or a desire to get back at them. No, you don't have to forget or excuse harmful behaviour, but you do need to decide whether you're going to hold on to it or let it go. If you're not ready to forgive, that's totally fine. Say so and be clear about what you need to get there. And if you don't think forgiveness is ever going to be on the table, that's okay too. That's a bigger conversation to have, and it might be easier with some professional support. To truly repair a relationship, you need to be clear about how you're feeling and only forgive someone when you are ready to let go of any emotions you've been hanging on to.

EXAMPLES OF REPAIR

Here's a list of some examples of repair that Billie and I each do in our respective relationships. These aren't meant to be rules that you have to follow so much as examples of practices and behaviours to give you some inspiration in your own life.

PRINCIPLE 8 — IMPROVE YOUR COMMUNICATION

Some things Anna and Luke do . . .

- **Clarify repair needs:** Ask if the other person wants a solution, support or space. Define what these look like for each of you.
- **Prioritize relationship maintenance:** Rather than letting things go unresolved, implement practices like weekly retrospectives (see p. 83) and monthly check-ins.
- **Don't forget to play:** After an argument, get silly and laugh with each other. For us, that's chasing each other around the house, having a boogie or being mischievous.
- **Keep it physical:** Experiment with different types of touch in different contexts and clarify what type of touch you need. For instance, affectionate touch, sensual touch, playful touch or calming touch.

Some things Billie and Seb do . . .

- **Respect different approaches:** If one partner prefers having a conversation immediately and the other needs time to digest, agree to pause the conversation and set a future date.
- **Use a trusted soundboard:** For difficult conversations, get support from a third party who can help you navigate with kindness. For us, that's our couples' coach Ellie.
- **Set up 'meetings' for long-term goals:** Once a month, we sync up on our long-term goals

and belief-based topics, like money, especially when planning for future decisions.
- **Surprise each other:** Rebuild trust and connection by leaving each other notes, planning surprise dates, picking up a favourite treat or doing something else that's thoughtful.

Improving communication in real life

The more we accept that difficult conversations are a part of life and we could all do with communicating better, the more empowered we become, both in and out of the bedroom. This is something Billie and I have worked on together, in our own lives, and with loads of women around the world. Like any skill, communication is one anyone can develop, and with practice and a little bit of patience, it's also one you're capable of mastering.

Here's how it went for me...

I wish I could say Adam and I learned to communicate well and were able to have the difficult conversations we needed, but we never did. Instead of resolving things, we kept avoiding talking about anything that was uncomfortable, sweeping it under the rug and pretending everything was fine. Eventually, all the things we left unsaid piled up so high, there was no longer any way of ignoring them. They showed up in passive-aggressive — and aggressive — comments, feelings of bitterness and resentment, and an overall sense of walking on eggshells around each other. We either had to open up or break up — we ended up calling it quits.

PRINCIPLE 8 – IMPROVE YOUR COMMUNICATION

There are a lot of reasons why Adam and I didn't work out, but the biggest one by far was our total inability to communicate. We avoided difficult conversations at all costs, until ironically, the cost was us. And if I'm being honest, this same pattern kept showing up across all my relationships, not just my romantic ones.

I used to struggle not only to communicate well, but to communicate at all.

Non-communicative me never developed the skills to express myself, and nor did I know what good communication looked like. More than that, non-communicative me didn't believe my needs were as important as other people's or even worth communicating in the first place.

What I did believe, and what formed a large part of my identity, was that being a 'good' person, like in my relationship with Adam, meant being supportive. Somewhere along the way, however, 'being supportive' got translated into putting other people's feelings and needs ahead of my own. Later, I'd learn that this was another variation of people-pleasing. It wasn't that I didn't want to speak up – I felt guilty for taking up space and I didn't know how. I was scared of getting it wrong, upsetting people or making a situation worse.

While I could get away with avoiding communication in my romantic relationships, there was no way I could avoid it at work. Although we didn't realize it at the time, starting Ferly was a real crash course for both Billie and I in how to communicate well (and how not to). It also forced both of us to get *real* comfortable talking about sex.

Fun fact: When Billie and I decided to build a business together, we'd only just met. People say the co-founder relationship is like a pseudo-marriage, and while it's not the healthiest analogy, it's also not entirely untrue. We moved fast. In a matter of months, we went from strangers to having our lives legally, financially, physically and emotionally bound to one another.

With all that, as partners, we quickly had to figure out how we were (and weren't) compatible. I liked structure, she preferred spontaneity. She liked doing things as a team, I liked doing things solo. I favoured cooperation, she favoured competition. Not only were we opposite personalities, but we also had opposite defaults when it came to conflict. She'd go into fight mode, I'd go into flight mode. I'd be passive-aggressive, she'd be aggressive. Of course, we didn't yet know this about each other because we didn't even know it about ourselves. Like a lot of committed relationships, we were trying to make it work and trying to build a future together, while also trying to figure out who the heck we were.

Eventually, as it did with Adam, all the unresolved stuff between Billie and I started to pile up. And also, like with Adam, we hit a point where we either had to commit to communicating better or accept that our relationship – and everything we were working to build – wouldn't last, at least not in a way that felt good. Luckily, unlike the average couple, we didn't wait six years before getting help. Instead, we started working with a coach to learn how to move through our relationship ruptures – and more importantly, to prioritize our relationship repair. We did this by appreciating our strengths and complementarities, as well as learning how to balance each other's weaknesses. Our coach also helped to guide us through difficult conversations until we developed the skills to handle them on our own.

It was during this work that I realized a lot of my communication issues came from my own lack of self-confidence and self-esteem, which particularly showed up as identity triggers – not only in my professional relationships but in my personal relationships too.

PRINCIPLE 8 – IMPROVE YOUR COMMUNICATION

A few months prior, I'd gone through my mental health breakdown and I was still very much rebuilding my sense of self. Before the breakdown, I hadn't believed my needs mattered. After the breakdown and my recovery, I had finally begun to see that, like everyone else, I was also worthy of love, respect and kindness, which meant holding space to communicate my needs.

To get better at managing my identity triggers, expressing my needs, and to feel more confident having difficult conversations, I started to build and practise different communication skills, applying a new one each month. These included: making and declining requests; using 'I' statements; jotting down my thoughts before sharing them; cutting back on overexplaining and over-apologizing; getting regular feedback from people I trusted; not multitasking or interrupting when I was listening; and reflecting back what I'd heard to make sure that I'd understood correctly.

The more confident a communicator I became outside of the bedroom, the better able I became at applying those same skills to my sex life.

A couple of years later, when Luke and I started dating, we spoke about building good communication habits and talking openly about sex from the get-go. We discussed what we liked, what we didn't like, and how we could make our sexual experiences better together. Because we both had experience with navigating desire discrepancies in our previous relationships, we also talked about the importance of how to keep up intimacy in low seasons and the importance of regular non-sexual touch. We're big believers in doing weekly relationship retros (see p. 83). For us, this is one of the most important ways to prevent rupture and prioritize ongoing repair.

When I compare non-communicative me, like how I was in my relationship with Adam, to where I am now, I almost don't recognize myself (in a good way). As someone who not only failed to communicate well, but to communicate at all, I'm proud of how I've improved and am still improving. I'm also proud of Luke and how we have committed to working through our communication challenges, even though we still get it wrong sometimes.

I now feel confident expressing my needs across various relationships in my life. I've also gotten better at giving and receiving feedback and managing my identity triggers, and I no longer avoid conflict. Sure, I still get a bit nervous or apprehensive when I have to have a difficult conversation, but I trust in myself to get through them. One of my biggest learnings has been that if you can communicate well in the bedroom and in your romantic relationships, which are some of the most intimate and vulnerable settings, you can communicate anywhere.

Being great at communication is a skill. Your goal isn't to be perfect, but to improve little by little each time – which, by reading this chapter, you've already started to do. Now that you know more about how to have a difficult conversation, how to navigate feedback and how to do relationship repair, you're well on your way to finding your power and getting not just what you want, but what you need.

In practice: Here's how to improve communication

Tool #1: *Identify and express your sexual needs*

Identifying and talking about our sexual needs can feel a bit uncomfortable but it doesn't have to. Think of

PRINCIPLE 8 – IMPROVE YOUR COMMUNICATION

these questions as conversation starters to help you and/or your partner get on the same page – kind of like having a personalized guidebook for your sex life. Answering them openly and honestly removes some of the guesswork and can help you feel more confident talking about sex and expressing your sexual needs.

MY SEXUAL NEEDS: CONVERSATION PROMPTS

1. My definition of pleasure is . . .
2. The environment I feel most comfortable having sex in is . . .
3. I'm curious to know more about or try . . .
4. A fantasy or romantic daydream I have is . . .
5. I think of masturbation and solo sex as . . .
6. Five things that make me more open to sex are . . .
7. Five things that make me not want to have sex are . . .
8. When it comes to initiating sex, I like . . .
9. What I want during foreplay is . . .
10. Three things that I enjoy during sex are . . .
11. Three things I don't enjoy during sex are . . .
12. Areas of my body that I want touched are . . .
13. Areas of my body that I don't want to be touched are . . .
14. The pace, pressure and types of touch I find most pleasurable are . . .
15. Sexual acts I am open to giving are . . .
16. Sexual acts I am open to receiving are . . .
17. My boundaries or hard limits are . . .

18. When it comes to using things like toys, props or porn, I . . .
19. Sex is 'done' when . . .
20. After sex, I want to . . .

Tool #2: Take stock of where you're at

To help you improve your communication and feel more confident when navigating feedback, we've created a reflection tool to help you to take stock of where you're at. To illustrate how it works, we've drawn on my fight with Luke as an example. You'll need a journal or a notebook to get started or you can download a template from www.turnyourselfon.co.

Here are your step-by-step instructions:

1. Start by copying out the three headings from each column in the table on p. 306. Once you have those, write down all the reflection prompts in the first column. Leave yourself plenty of room to answer them in columns two ('My Reflections') and three ('My Future Strategies').
2. Think about a recent conflict or misunderstanding you've had, with a partner, a family member, a friend or a co-worker. This will be your starting example.
3. Responding to the reflection prompts in the left-hand column, fill out details of what happened during that conflict in the 'My Reflections' column.

4. Once you've filled out the 'My Reflections' column, take a moment to think about what you've learned about yourself and what insights you've gained.
5. Drawing on these insights and learnings, come up with ideas for how you might handle future conversations differently or better. In the 'My Future Strategies' column, write 1–3 strategies down that could help you communicate better in the future.
6. Keep your answers somewhere safe, and repeat this exercise after any future conflicts.
7. Look back at your answers over time and see if you can pick out any patterns. Pay attention to which strategies work (and don't work) for you.

Reflection Prompts	My Reflections	My Future Strategies
What happened? Describe the situation as it factually occurred	*Luke and I were making dinner, I brought up future career decisions and kids, Luke made a comment about responsibility, I got defensive . . .*	*Consider the timing and context of when I bring up a big topic*
How did this make me feel? Describe how you felt	*Misunderstood, confused and guilty*	*Express my feelings so they don't burst, block or leak*
What thoughts did I have? Describe any thoughts or assumptions you made	*I need to fix things and make sure Luke's not upset*	*Honour Luke's request for time*
How was my sense of self challenged? Reflect on how this challenged your identity or your beliefs	*Independence is important to me, and I felt this was threatened when . . .*	*Manage my all-or-nothing thinking*

Reflection Prompts	My Reflections	My Future Strategies
What triggered me? Identify things that you had a strong emotional or psychological response to (e.g. words, behaviours, setting)	*When Luke said 'It's fine' and didn't want to talk....*	*Share my triggers with Luke so we can....*
What did I do well? Describe positive behaviours	*I tried to initiate a conversation and to talk about....*	*Keep encouraging us to talk about issues as they happen*
What could I have done differently or better? Describe negative or unhelpful behaviours	*Not gone straight into 'solving mode' and given Luke some space to process....*	*Agree to pause a conversation and come back to it later*

Tool #3: Take a forgiveness walk

We all know that sometimes relationships need a little TLC, and what better way to patch things up and do a bit of relationship repair than with a forgiveness walk? This activity isn't just about getting some fresh air and stretching your legs, it's also a powerful way to physically and symbolically move forward from past hurts while engaging in heartfelt conversation and mutual forgiveness. Some parts might feel a little cheesy and that's okay – they're worth it.

What you'll need:

- Paper and pens (opt for biodegradable where possible to keep it green)
- A lighter or matches, and a small metal container or mug that you can burn paper in
- A peaceful, quiet walking route

Step 1: Prep time

- **Gather your supplies:** Make sure you have your paper, pens, metal container and lighter.
- **Pick your path:** Choose a serene route that feels right for a reflective walk, with a natural spot like a viewpoint or a bench to safely carry out your burning ritual.

PRINCIPLE 8 — IMPROVE YOUR COMMUNICATION

Step 2: Write down your grievances

- Before you hit the road, take a moment to each jot down any grievances on your individual pieces of paper. These could be things you're ready to forgive or seeking forgiveness for.

Step 3: Go on your forgiveness walk

- Begin your walk together, keeping the vibe calm and reflective. Discuss what you've written down, aiming to share feelings openly but gently. Focus on taking turns listening and sharing.

Step 4: Let it go

- At a meaningful point during your walk — maybe halfway or at a special spot or after grabbing a coffee — place the papers in the metal container or mug, light them up and watch them burn, symbolizing the letting-go of past issues.
- During this ritual, share a moment of silence, look each other in the eyes for a few seconds or say some words of affirmation to mark the release.

Step 5: Time to forgive

- After your release ritual, openly offer forgiveness to each other. This can be through specific statements like 'I forgive you for . . .' or more spontaneous expressions based on how the release made you feel.

Step 6: Wrap it up and reconnect

- As you continue your walk, talk about how the ritual felt and discuss ways to prevent future grievances and how you might improve your communication going forward.
- Finish your walk with a gesture that brings you closer. This might be a hug, holding hands, a kiss or verbal expressions of gratitude and appreciation.

Look back to look forward

Take 1–2 minutes to reflect and answer the following questions:

1. How am I communicating well?
2. How am I not communicating well?
3. What's one action I'm going to start, stop or continue NOW to be better at communicating in my life?

If you'd like to dive deeper, we've hooked you up with some great resources and downloadable templates at www.turnyourselfon.co.

PRINCIPLE 8 – IMPROVE YOUR COMMUNICATION

Cement your learnings

- Of all the conversations we have, talking about sex still remains one of the most taboo. That's why expressing yourself sexually is a great place to start practising how to improve your communication. If you can master it in your most intimate and vulnerable settings, you can master it anywhere.
- When it comes to improving our sex lives and relationships, communication is the most important skill we can develop. It is the single biggest predictor of both sexual and relationship satisfaction, as well as whether a relationship is likely to last.
- Communication involves two roles: giver and receiver. We take on both roles simultaneously, and there's a lot of room for error and misunderstanding between them, which is what makes communication so tricky.
- When you have a difficult conversation, you're having three conversations at the same time: 'What Happened?', 'Feelings' and 'Identity' (see p. 279). Being aware of each of these can help you communicate more effectively.
- To receive feedback well, you need to manage your triggers. Three common ones are truth, relationship and identity triggers (see p. 286).
- A helpful framework for giving feedback is the Situation, Behaviour, Impact and

Action (SBIA) framework (see p. 291). This can help avoid criticizing and defending behaviours.
- Healthy relationships need reconnection (repair) after disconnection (rupture). How you repair is individual but generally includes a conversation where you share your feelings, apologize and forgive (see p. 295).

Bonus reads

- Douglas Stone, Bruce Patton and Sheila Heen, *Difficult Conversations: How to Discuss What Matters Most*
- Douglas Stone and Sheila Heen, *Thanks for the Feedback: The Science and Art of Receiving Feedback Well*
- Kate Murphy, *You're Not Listening: What You're Missing and Why It Matters*
- Oren Jay Sofer, *Say What You Mean: A Mindful Approach to Nonviolent Communication*
- Marshall B. Rosenberg, PhD, *Nonviolent Communication: A Language of Life: Life-Changing Tools for Healthy Relationships*
- Chris Voss, *Never Split the Difference: Negotiating As If Your Life Depended On It*

Conclusion

'Who are *you*?' said the Caterpillar.

This was not an encouraging opening for a conversation. Alice replied, rather shyly, 'I – I hardly know, sir, just at present – at least I know who I *was* when I got up this morning, but I think I must have been changed several times since then...'[1]

Alright not-actually-Alice, you're here, you've made it!

You tumbled down the rabbit hole of self-discovery. You explored the wondrous (and sometimes bewildering) world of your own sexuality, and each principle in this book has been a new door to unlocking, exploring and revealing insights about yourself. Congratulations on walking right on through. Now, you're returning from Wonderland and coming back to the real world...

As we're nearing the end of this part of your journey, let's take a moment to reflect on where you were and where you are now – how *you* may have changed several times since the beginning of this book. Close your eyes and picture your sex life. Think about some of the stuff that might come with it – for example intimacy, desire, pleasure, novelty, confidence and communication.

Now, think about where you're currently at and how you might make your sex life better. How confident are you, on a scale from 1 to 10, in the steps you need to take to improve it? With 1 being 'Um, no idea' and 10 being 'Totally got this'.

Got your number? Great! Hold it in your head.

Now, remember that number you scribbled down when you first picked up this book?

Go ahead and check it out.

Has it changed? If so, why?

There's no right or wrong answer here. We're all on journeys of self-discovery, especially when it comes to our sexual selves. Knowing what turns you on – both in bed and in life – is about as personal as it gets. This book isn't a cheat sheet, it's more like a trusty compass, guiding you to transform your relationship with sex, your partner and, most importantly, yourself. As you emerge from this rabbit hole, you'll probably find yourself tumbling down another. That's the beauty of our sexual selves and the thrill of self-discovery – we're constantly growing and evolving. In the same way our relationships and lives change, our sexualities change too.

Cement your learnings

Sometimes it can be hard to keep track of all that change or those light-bulb moments, especially over time. To help you make sense of everything you've learned so far, here's a recap of all the stops you've visited, the discoveries you've made and the tools you've picked up over the course of this book . . .

CONCLUSION

First up, you **asserted your agency**. You've been the captain of your own ship, steering through the seas of decision-making and holding your own. Remember how you explored boundaries like Goldilocks? Not too porous, not too rigid, but just right? And how about the moment you realized consent is more than the absence of a 'no', but freely and readily choosing to participate? You've already practised asserting your agency by identifying your boundary style, setting boundaries and using tools like the Eisenhower Matrix to make more empowered decisions (see p. 46). How's that for taking command?

Then, there was **balancing your power**. You learned power isn't only about wielding influence over others, but also about fostering 'power to' and 'power with'. You've spotted red, amber and green flag behaviours, from the baddies like gaslighting to the goodies like taking responsibility and expressing gratitude. You've mapped power dynamics, done weekly retrospectives and even conducted a joy audit to discover what turns you on in life (see p. 85).

After that, you stopped at a tea party, but this time the Mad Hatter was dishing out a three-tiered layered cake **built from your self-confidence, self-esteem and self-efficacy**. Did we just take the metaphor too far? Probably, but we're nerds at heart so we're here for it. In this chapter, you saw how each layer plays a crucial role in shaping your sense of self and making you feel powerful both in and out of the bedroom. You reframed your beliefs, challenged your cognitive distortions and manifested your future, turning your dreams into reality, one confident step at a time (see p. 114).

Cultivating your intimacy is about way more than having sex. It is about diving inwards, understanding what intimacy means to you and building connections deeper than the Mariana Trench. Chapter 4 explored how your attachment style shapes your relationships and you discovered social connection is a drive. Likewise, how intimacy is a need, not a nice-to-have. Through tools like the intimate needs inventory and practising gratitude (see p. 150), you've been nurturing connections that are as enriching as they are essential.

Embracing your desire took you for a spin as you uncovered that desire is a motivation not a drive, and that it can be responsive too. You learned about the dual-control model, balancing your sexual accelerator and brakes, arousal non-concordance and the mystery of why your body and mind can feel out of sync. Your desire inventory, body mapping and touch menu have been tools for tuning out the noise of the world (see p. 180), and zeroing in on what turns you on.

Of course, understanding desire is one thing, but if you want to access it, you need to **honour your health** too. Your journey into your nervous system was a reminder that self-care isn't selfish, it's essential. You delved into the world of mental health, and discovered how rest and play can recharge your batteries. Breathwork, progressive muscle relaxation and uncovering your unique play personalities (see p. 221) are all tools you've now added to your self-care toolkit.

Once you learned how to take care of yourself from stress to rest-and-digest, you created a context

CONCLUSION

that allowed you to **prioritize your pleasure**. You discovered pleasure is so much more than the Big O. On your adventure through your own sensual Wonderland, you explored eroticism, mindfulness and fantasy, learning to tune in to your body and savour experiences. Crafting erotic fantasies, doing arousal awareness meditations, self-pleasuring and experimenting with partnered play (see p. 257) have been a few ways you've started putting pleasure front and centre.

Finally, you've worked to **improve your communication** and to master the art of both giving and receiving. You've navigated difficult conversations, feedback and relationship repair, and ensuring that your voice is heard, your triggers are managed and your desires are met. Identifying and expressing your sexual needs and using frameworks like SBIA (see p. 291) have been steps towards becoming a communication pro.

Looking back at it, you've done a lot!

Billie and I hope that over the last eight chapters, you've come to realize that this is about so much more than having better sex. It's about understanding that your sexuality – whatever it may be – is an inherent part of who you are and how you show up in the world. Sex isn't just something you do, it's something you can use. It's a powerful tool for your own self-discovery, one that is as mental and emotional as it is physical. In getting to know your sexual self, you have connected with your own inner erotic guide and embraced a fuller and more authentic version of you. Want proof? Here it is . . .

Look back to look forward: What's next?

We told you from the get-go, this book is like your trusty toolbox – it's not meant to be read, it's meant to be used. So let's use it. Let's put it all together and explore the future 'you' and the 'you' you are already becoming. It's time to peek inside your mind, body and heart one last time before we go. Given that it's your last hurrah, we've tweaked it a bit and added a few more questions to get you thinking about what's next.

> Take 10–15 minutes (or as long as you'd like) to reflect and answer the following questions either here or in your trusty notebook:
>
> LOOK BACK
>
> Over the course of this book, **my top three biggest learnings have been** . . .
>
> What I'm **doing well** is . . .
>
> What I'm **not doing so well** is . . .

CONCLUSION

Dear younger me . . . **if I could go back and tell you one thing**, it would be . . .

As I look back on our journey together, **I want you to know** . . .

LOOK FORWARD

My **definition of 'good sex'** is . . .

When I think about improving my sex life going forward, **the words that most describe how I'm feeling are** . . .

The aspect of my sex life that **I would most like to continue working on is** . . .

Dear future me . . . (Imagine yourself twelve months from now and write a note to your future self about how you're feeling and what's going to be different in a year. For good measure, add in 1–3 positive things to hype yourself up.)

WHAT'S NEXT

What are three actions I can take to continue my journey? (Make sure your goals are specific, measurable, achievable, realistic and time-bound.)

Tip: Compare your answers to where you were at when you started. Remember those three questions we asked on page 4? Go back to what you wrote down when you first picked up this book.

If you'd like to dive deeper, we've hooked you up with some great resources and downloadable templates at www.turnyourselfon.co.

Pause for a second and give yourself a big hug. Actually do it though – take a moment to celebrate your wins. Look at you, emerging from your journey

CONCLUSION

of self-discovery, transformed and more powerful than ever. You're not the same person you were when you first cracked open this book – the proof is in the pudding. You're wiser, more equipped and ready to embrace the wonders of not only your sexuality, but your entire life. You've turned the pages, soaked up the learnings and most importantly you've already embarked on the journey to becoming a more empowered version of you, both in and out of the bedroom.

This is a book for any woman who wants to have a better sex life.

It's also a book of self-discovery.

We've said it before and we'll say it again, great sex starts solo (louder for the people at the back!). The knowledge and tools you've gathered over the course of this book are yours for keeps. As long as you're interested in having great sex and a great life, this book will continue to be your guide, hopefully for years to come. By diving into these eight principles and applying them to your life, you've now got the blueprint you need to turn yourself on and have a healthier, more confident and more pleasurable life in everything you do.

Not only do you have the knowledge and the tools to do just that, you've also built something bigger: connection. Connection to yourself, to us and to the many other women who are on a similar journey. At the beginning of this book, we spoke about shame and how shame loves to live in the shadows. By bringing light to our stories, and those of other women throughout these chapters, we hope you know that whatever your own story might be, it can always be rewritten. It's up to you to choose how it's told and how it will unfold.

If you're going to take one thing away from this book, let it be this: the most important relationship you'll ever have is the one you have with yourself. Go forward by giving yourself permission to turn yourself on and lean into your aliveness, to nurture that connection with yourself and the world around you, and to cultivate the fullest and most powerful version of you. Now, go get it.

xx Anna + Billie

Will you help us empower more women?

Here are three meaningful ways you can support and drive change:

1. If you liked this book, would you mind writing a review on Amazon? Even a short one helps to reassure and encourage future readers, and it would mean a lot to us.
2. If someone you know is going through a rough patch with intimacy or is feeling a bit stuck in their life, please send them this book. You can gift them a copy or direct them to www.turnyourselfon.co – whichever you choose is fine by us.
3. If you want to continue on your journey, connect with us and this community, and get access to bonus material, downloadable resources and templates, check out www.turnyourselfon.co for more!

Here's to you and your adventure cultivating a healthy, confident and pleasurable life. Time to turn yourself on . . .

Lots of love,
Anna & Billie

Acknowledgements

We'll keep it short and sweet...

To all the women who've been a part of Ferly, and who have trusted us with their own journeys, thank you. To our beta readers – especially Stephanie, Esme, Sara, Lydia, Elena Jerilee, Darlene, Alita, Elise, Masa, Lucy, Eleanor, Henrietta, Julianne and Elaine – thank you for your time, honesty and incredible feedback. Each and every one of you made this book happen.

To Amy McWalters and the crew at Penguin, thank you for encouraging us to be rebellious, shake things up and stay true to who we are. This is a phenomenal work of collaboration and goes way beyond our own efforts.

To our investors, and especially Julia Hawkins and Check Warner, thank you for believing in us from day one. We couldn't have built Ferly without you and your unbelievable commitment and dedication to paving the way and creating opportunities for other women.

To our advisors – especially the brilliant Kate Moyle, Dr Karen Gurney and Dr Lori Brotto – thank you for continuously offering insights, learnings and support with active minds and open arms. Here's to the many practitioners and researchers improving science and healthcare for women around the world.

ACKNOWLEDGEMENTS

To our own communities, the girls and the people in our lives who have inspired us, challenged us and kept us whole – thank you. You've been with us for years – through the laughs, the cries, the good, the bad and everything in between – and so much of who we are, we are because of you. Here's to you and to many more years to come.

To Jeff and Mark, who've been our own ride-or-dies, and to Lynn, Mary Ann, Janet and Eugene, for more than words can ever say.

Thank you.

And to each other. To a love story that has been unlike any other.

Notes

A Note from Billie

1 Brown, B. (2010), 'The Power of Vulnerability [Video]', TEDx Houston Conference.

Introduction

1 Frederick, D. A., John, H. K. S., Garcia, J. R., and Lloyd, E. A. (2018), 'Differences in Orgasm Frequency Among Gay, Lesbian, Bisexual, and Heterosexual Men and Women in a U.S. National Sample', *Archives of Sexual Behavior*, 47(1), 273–88.
2 Brown, B. (2012), *Daring Greatly: How the Courage to Be Vulnerable Transforms the Way We Live, Love, Parent and Lead*, Penguin Publishing Group.
3 Ibid.
4 Kross, E., Berman, M. G., Mischel, W., Smith, E. E., and Wager, T. D. (2011), 'Social Rejection Shares Somatosensory Representations with Physical Pain', *Proceedings of the National Academy of Sciences of the United States of America*, 108(15), 6270–75; Boring, B. L., Walsh, K. T., Nanavaty, N., and Mathur, V. A. (2021), 'Shame Mediates the Relationship Between Pain Invalidation and Depression', *Frontiers in Psychology*, 12(743584); Bastin, C., Harrison,

B. J., Davey, C. G., Moll, J., and Whittle, S. (2016), 'Feelings of Shame, Embarrassment and Guilt and their Neural Correlates: A Systematic Review', *Neuroscience & Biobehavioral Reviews*, 71, 455–71; Piretti, L., Pappaianni, E., Garbin, C., Rumiati, R. I., Job, R., and Grecucci, A. (2023), 'The Neural Signatures of Shame, Embarrassment, and Guilt: A Voxel-Based Meta-Analysis on Functional Neuroimaging Studies', *Brain Sciences*, 13(4), 559.
5 World Health Organization (2006a), 'Defining Sexual Health: Report of a Technical Consultation on Sexual Health 28–31 January 2002, Geneva', *Sexual Health Document Series*, World Health Organization, Geneva.

Principle 1 – Assert Your Agency

1 Kabeer, N. (1999), 'Resources, Agency, Achievements: Reflections on the Measurement of Women's Empowerment', *Development and Change*, 30, 435–64; Sen, A. (1985), 'Well-being, Agency and Freedom: The Dewey Lectures 1984', *Journal of Philosophy*, 82(4), 169–221.
2 United Nations Women (2023), Facts and Figures, Women's Leadership and Political Participation.
3 United Nations Children's Fund (2022), Female Genital Mutilation (FGM).
4 King, P. (2020), *Establishing Boundaries: How to Protect Yourself, Become Assertive, Take Back Control, and Set Yourself Free*, Independently Published.
5 Rape Crisis England and Wales (2021), Rape and Sexual Assault Statistics (from the UK Office for National Statistics).

6 Katz, J., and Tirone, V. (2020), 'When Do Motives to Sexually Please a Male Partner Benefit Women's Own Sexual Agency?', *Sex Roles*, 82, 336–44.
7 Ibid.
8 Kennedy, B. (2024), 'Protocols for Excellent Parenting and Improving Relationships of all Kinds', *The Huberman Lab*, podcast episode 165, 16 February 2024.

Principle 2 – Balance Your Power

1 Farrell, A. K., Simpson, J. A., and Rothman, A. J. (2015), 'The Relationship Power Inventory: Development and Validation', *Personal Relationships*, 22, 387–413.
2 NATSAL-3. (2012), 'Sexual Attitudes and Lifestyles in Britain: Highlights from Natsal-3' [infographic].
3 Körner, R., and Schütz, A. (2021), 'Power in Romantic Relationships: How Positional and Experienced Power are Associated with Relationship Quality', *Journal of Social and Personal Relationships*, 38(9), 2653–77.
4 Pew Research (2008), 'Women Call the Shots at Home; Public Mixed on Gender Roles in Jobs'.
5 Pansardi, P., and Bindi, M. (2021), 'The New Concepts of Power? Power-Over, Power-To and Power-With', *Journal of Political Power*, 14(1), 51–71.
6 Office for National Statistics (2021), 'Sexual Offences Victim Characteristics, England and Wales: Year Ending March 2020'.
7 Amnesty International (2022), 'The Never-Ending Maze: Continued Failure to Protect Indigenous Women from Violence in the USA', May 17, 2022, AMR 51/5485/2022.

8 Ujima (2018), 'Black Women and Sexual Assault: Statistics of Black Women and Sexual Assault', The National Center on Violence Against Women in the Black Community.
9 Bryant-Davis, T., and Ocampo, C. (2005), 'The Trauma of Racism: Implications for Counseling, Research and Education', *The Counseling Psychologist*, 33, 574–8; Gómez, J. M. (2020), 'Black Women and Girls & #MeToo: Rape, Cultural Betrayal, and Healing', *Sex Roles: A Journal of Research*, 82, 1–12.
10 Fishbane, M. D. (2011), 'Facilitating Relational Empowerment in Couple Therapy', *Family Process*, 50(3), 337–52.
11 Pansardi and Bindi (2021); Allen, A. (1998), 'Rethinking Power', *Hypatia*, 13(1), 21–40.
12 Fishbane, M. D. (2011), 'Facilitating Relational Empowerment in Couple Therapy', *Family Process*, 50(3), 337–52.
13 Bates, L. (2020), *Men Who Hate Women: From Incels to Pickup Artists*, Simon and Schuster.
14 National Domestic Violence Hotline (2021), 'What Is Gaslighting?', https://thehotline.org/resources/what-is-gaslighting/, adapted from Tracy, N. (2021), 'Gaslighting Definition, Techniques and Being Gaslighted', Healthyplace.
15 Sweet, P. L. (2022), 'Understanding Gaslighting', *Scientific American*, 327(4).
16 Gottman, J., and Silver, N. (2015), *The Seven Principles for Making Marriage Work: A Practical Guide from the Country's Foremost Relationship Expert*, Harmony Books.
17 Ibid.
18 Gottman, J. M. (1994), *What Predicts Divorce? The Relationship Between Marital Processes and Marital Outcomes*, Lawrence Erlbaum Associates.

Principle 3 – Build Your Self-Confidence

1 Kay, K., and Shipman, C. (2014), *The Confidence Code: The Science and Art of Self-Assurance – What Women Should Know*, HarperBusiness.
2 Babcock, L., and Laschever, S. (2021), *Women Don't Ask: Negotiation and the Gender Divide*, Princeton University Press.
3 Ehrlinger, J., and Dunning, D. (2003), 'How Chronic Self-Views Influence (and Potentially Mislead) Estimates of Performance', *Journal of Personality and Social Psychology*, 84(1), 5–17.
4 The Confidence Code for Girls x Ypulse (2018), 'The Confidence Code for Girls: The Confidence Collapse and Why it Matters for the Next Gen'.
5 Dove (2017), 'The 2017 Dove Global Girls Beauty and Confidence Report'.
6 Bachman, J. G., O'Malley, P. M., Freedman-Doan, P., Trzesniewski, K. H., and Donnellan, M. B. (2011), 'Adolescent Self-Esteem: Differences by Race/Ethnicity, Gender, and Age', *Self and Identity*, 10(4), 445–73.
7 Burns, K. M., Burns, N. R., and Ward, L. (2016), 'Confidence – More a Personality or Ability Trait? It Depends on How it is Measured: A Comparison of Young and Older Adults', *Frontiers in Psychology*, 7, 518.
8 Lefkowitz, E. S., et al. (2014), 'How Gendered Attitudes Relate to Women's and Men's Sexual Behaviors and Beliefs', *Sexuality & Culture*, 18, 833–46; Katz, J., and Tirone, V. (2020), 'When Do Motives to Sexually Please a Male Partner Benefit Women's Own Sexual Agency?', *Sex Roles*, 82, 336–44.

9 Bleidorn, W., Arslan, R. C., Denissen, J. J., Rentfrow, P. J., Gebauer, J. E., Potter, J., and Gosling, S. D. (2016), 'Age and Gender Differences in Self-Esteem – A Cross-Cultural Window', *Journal of Personality and Social Psychology*, 111(3), 396–410.
10 Bandura, A. (1997), *Self-Efficacy: The Exercise of Control*, W H Freeman/Times Books/Henry Holt & Co.
11 Branden, N. (1995), *The Six Pillars of Self-Esteem: The Definitive Work on Self-Esteem by the Leading Pioneer in the Field*, Bantam.

Principle 4 – Cultivate Your Intimacy

1 Gottman and Silver (2015); Simpson, J. A., Rholes, W. S., and Phillips, D. (1996), 'Conflict in Close Relationships: An Attachment Perspective', *Journal of Personality and Social Psychology*, 71(5), 899–914; Levine, A., and Heller, R. S. F. (2012), *Attached: The New Science of Adult Attachment and How it Can Help You Find – and Keep – Love*, Penguin Random House.
2 Yoo, H., Bartle-Haring, S., Day, R. D., and Gangamma, R. (2014), 'Couple Communication, Emotional and Sexual Intimacy, and Relationship Satisfaction', *Journal of Sex and Marital Therapy*, 40(4), 275–93; Doss, B. D., Simpson, L. E., and Christensen, A. (2004), 'Why Do Couples Seek Marital Therapy?', *Professional Psychology: Research and Practice*, 35(6), 608–14.
3 Office for National Statistics (2017), 'Divorces in England and Wales' [statistical bulletin].
4 Basson, R. (2000), 'The Female Sexual Response: A Different Model', *Journal of Sex and Marital Therapy*, 26(1), 51–65; Stephenson, K. R., and Meston, C. M. (2010),

'When are Sexual Difficulties Distressing for Women? The Selective Protective Value of Intimate Relationships', *Journal of Sexual Medicine*, 7(11), 3683–94; Rubin, H., and Campbell, L. (2012), 'Day-To-Day Changes in Intimacy Predict Heightened Relationship Passion, Sexual Occurrence, and Sexual Satisfaction: A Dyadic Diary Analysis', *Social Psychological and Personality Science*, 3, 224–31; Muise, A., Giang, E., and Impett, E. A. (2014), 'Post Sex Affectionate Exchanges Promote Sexual and Relationship Satisfaction', *Archives of Sexual Behavior*, 43(7), 1391–1402; Birnbaum, G. E., Reis, H. T., Mizrahi, M., Kanat-Maymon, Y., Sass, O., and Granovski-Milner, C. (2016), 'Intimately Connected: The Importance of Partner Responsiveness for Experiencing Sexual Desire', *Journal of Personality and Social Psychology*, 111, 53–64.

5 Van Lankveld, J., Jacobs, N., Thewissen, V., Dewitte, M., and Verboon, P. (2018), 'The Associations of Intimacy and Sexuality in Daily Life: Temporal Dynamics and Gender Effects Within Romantic Relationships', *Journal of Social and Personal Relationships*, 35(4), 557–76; Brown, J. (2021), The Potent Cocktail of Love, Intimacy, Sex, and Power: An Assessment Pyramid for Couples Therapy', *Sexual and Relationship Therapy*, 36(4), 413–37; Yoo, H., Bartle-Haring, S., Day, R. D., and Gangamma, R. (2014), 'Couple Communication, Emotional and Sexual Intimacy, and Relationship Satisfaction', *Journal of Sex and Marital Therapy*, 40(4), 275–93; Pascoal, P. M., Narciso, I. S. B., and Pereira, N.M. (2014), 'What is Sexual Satisfaction? Thematic Analysis of Lay People's Definitions', *Journal of Sex Research*, 51(1), 22–30.

6 Schnarch, D. (2009), *Intimacy & Desire: Awaken the Passion in Your Relationship*, Beaufort Books.

7 Birnbaum, G. E., Reis, H. T., Mikulincer, M., Gillath, O., and Orpaz, A. (2006), 'When Sex is More Than Just Sex: Attachment Orientations, Sexual Experience, and Relationship Quality', *Journal of Personality and Social Psychology*, 91(5), 929.
8 Levine and Heller (2012).
9 Birnbaum et al. (2006).
10 Schnarch, D. (2009), *Intimacy & Desire: Awaken the Passion in Your Relationship*, Beaufort Books.
11 Levine and Heller, (2012).
12 Lee, C. R., Chen, A., and Tye, K. M. (2021), 'The Neural Circuitry of Social Homeostasis: Consequences of Acute Versus Chronic Social Isolation', *Cell*, 184(6), 1500–16; Matthew, G. A., and Tye, K. M. (2019), 'Neutral Mechanisms of Social Homeostasis', *Annals of the New York Academy of Sciences*, 1457(1), 5–25.
13 Lee, Chen and Tye (2021); Matthew and Tye (2019).
14 Mushtaq, R., Shoib, S., Shah, T., and Mushtaq, S. (2014), 'Relationship Between Loneliness, Psychiatric Disorders and Physical Health? A Review on the Psychological Aspects of Loneliness', *Journal of Clinical and Diagnostic Research*, 8(9), WE01–04.
15 Czyżowska, D., Gurba, E., Czyżowska, N., Kalus, A., Sitnik-Warchulska, K., and Izydorczyk, B. (2019), 'Selected Predictors of the Sense of Intimacy in Relationships of Young Adults', *International Journal of Environmental Research and Public Health*, 16(22), 4447; Cacioppo, J., and Cacioppo, S. (2014), 'Social Relationships and Health: The Toxic Effects of Perceived Social Isolation', *Social and Personality Psychology Compass*, 8(2), 58–72; Haggerty, B. B., Bradbury, T. N., and Karney, B. R. (2022), 'The Disconnected Couple: Intimate

Relationships in the Context of Social Isolation', *Current Opinion in Psychology*, 43(2022), 24–9.
16 Johnson, S. M. (2019), *Attachment Theory in Practice: Emotionally Focused Therapy (EFT) With Individuals, Couples, and Families*, The Guilford Press, 6.
17 Perel, E., and Miller, M. A. (2023), 'Our Comfort with Intimacy Has a Lot to Do with These 7 Verbs', https://estherperel.com/blog/language-of-intimacy-and-7-verbs.
18 Fox, G. R., Kaplan, J., Damasio, H., and Damasio, A. (2015), 'Neural Correlates of Gratitude', *Frontiers in Psychology*, 6, 1491; Hazlett, L. I., Moieni, M., Irwin, M. R., Haltom, K. E. B., Jevtic, I., Meyer, M. L., Breen, E. C., Cole, S. W., and Eisenberger, N. I. (2021), 'Exploring Neural Mechanisms of the Health Benefits of Gratitude in Women: A Randomized Controlled Trial', *Brain, Behavior, and Immunity*, 95, 444–53; Woody, C. A., Ferrari, A. J., Siskind, D. J., Whiteford, H. A., and Harris, M. G. (2017), 'A Systematic Review and Meta-Regression of the Prevalence and Incidence of Perinatal Depression', *Journal of Affective Disorders*, 219, 86–92; Algoe, S. B., Gable, S. L., and Maisel, N. C. (2010), 'It's the Little Things: Everyday Gratitude as a Booster Shot for Romantic Relationships', *Personal Relationships*, 17(2), 217–33.
19 Fox et al. (2015).

Principle 5 – Embrace Your Desire

1 Goldner, V. (2004), 'Review Essay: Attachment and Eros: Opposed or Synergistic?', *Psychoanalytic Dialogues*, 14(3), 381–96.

2 NATSAL-3. (2012).
3 Brotto, L. A. (2018), *Better Sex Through Mindfulness: How Women Can Cultivate Desire*, Greystone Books.
4 Gurney, K. (2020), *Mind the Gap: The Truth About Desire, and How to Futureproof Your Sex Life*, Headline Home.
5 Freud, S. (1905), 'Three Essays on the Theory of Sexuality', *The Standard Edition of the Complete Psychological Works of Sigmund Freud*, Volume VII (1901–1905): *A Case of Hysteria, Three Essays on Sexuality and Other Works*, 123–46.
6 Nagoski, E. (2024), *Come Together: The Science (and Art!) of Creating Lasting Sexual Connections*, Penguin Random House, 3.
7 Basson, R. (2000), 'The Female Sexual Response: A Different Model', *Journal of Sex and Marital Therapy*, 26(1), 51–65.
8 Ibid., 51–65; Brotto, L. A. (2018), *Better Sex Through Mindfulness: How Women Can Cultivate Desire*, Greystone Books.
9 Gurney (2020); Basson, R. (2000), 'The Female Sexual Response: A Different Model', *Journal of Sex and Marital Therapy*, 26(1), 51–65; Brotto (2018); Nagoski (2015).
10 Bancroft, J., and Janssen, E. (2000), 'The Dual Control Model of Male Sexual Response: A Theoretical Approach to Centrally Mediated Erectile Dysfunction', *Neuroscience Biobehavior Review*, 24(5), 571–9.
11 Nagoski, E. (2015), *Come As You Are: The Surprising New Science that Will Transform Your Sex Life*, Simon and Schuster.
12 Ibid.
13 Herbenick, D., Mullinax, M., and Mark, K. (2014), 'Sexual Desire Discrepancy as a Feature, not a Bug, of Long-Term Relationships: Women's Self-Reported

Strategies for Modulating Sexual Desire', *Journal of Sexual Medicine*, 11(9), 2196–2206.

14 Prescott, H., and Khan, I. (2020), 'Medicinal Plants/Herbal Supplements as Female Aphrodisiacs: Does Any Evidence Exist to Support their Inclusion or Potential in the Treatment of FSD?', *Journal of Ethnopharmacology*, 251, 112464.

15 Herbenick, D., Mullinax, M., and Mark, K. (2014), 'Sexual Desire Discrepancy as a Feature, not a Bug, of Long-Term Relationships: Women's Self-Reported Strategies for Modulating Sexual Desire', *Journal of Sexual Medicine*, 11(9), 2196–2206.

16 Nagoski (2024).

17 Perel, E. (2007), *Mating in Captivity: Unlocking Erotic Intelligence*, HarperCollins, 25.

18 Herbenick, D. (2009), *Because It Feels Good: A Woman's Guide to Sexual Pleasure and Satisfaction*, Rodale.

19 Chivers, M. L., Rieger, G., Latty, E., and Bailey, J. M. (2004), 'A Sex Difference in the Specificity of Sexual Arousal', *Psychological Science*, 15(11), 736–44.

20 Brotto (2018).

Principle 6 – Honour Your Health

1 Hawkins, M. A. (2022), *The Power of Boredom: Why Boredom is Essential for Creating a Meaningful Life*, Cold Noodle Creative.

2 Mental Health Foundation (2018), 'Stress Statistics: Results of Our 2018 Study', https://mentalhealth.org.uk/explore-mental-health/statistics/stress-statistics.

3 American Psychiatric Association (2022), 'Anxiety Disorders', *Diagnostic and Statistical Manual of Mental Disorders*,

5th ed., 215–31; American Psychiatric Association (2022), 'Depression: What is Depression?', https://psychiatry.org/patients-families/depression/what-is-depression; World Health Organization (2023), 'Fact Sheets: Depressive Disorder (Depression)', https://who.int/news-room/fact-sheets/detail/depression; Woody, C. A., Ferrari, A. J., Siskind, D. J., Whiteford, H. A., and Harris, M. G. (2017), 'A Systematic Review and Meta-Regression of the Prevalence and Incidence of Perinatal Depression', *Journal of Affective Disorders*, 219, 86–92.

4 American Psychiatric Association (2017), 'Mental Health Disparities: LGBTQ', https://psychiatry.org/getmedia/552df1c0-57f2-4489-88fa-432182ce815a/mental-health-facts-for-LGBTQ.pdf; Marlay, M., File, T., and Scherer, Z. (2022), 'LGBT Adults Report Anxiety, Depression at All Ages – Mental Health Struggles Higher Among LGBT Adults Than Non-LGBT Adults in All Age Groups', United States Census Bureau.

5 O'Loughlin, J. I., Rellini, A. H., and Brotto, L. A. (2020), 'How Does Childhood Trauma Impact Women's Sexual Desire? Role of Depression, Stress, and Cortisol', *Journal of Sex Research*, 57(7), 836–47; Brotto (2018); Brotto, L. A., Basson, R., Grabovac, A., Chivers, M., Zdaniuk, B., Bodnar, T., and Weinberg, J. (2024), 'Impact of Mindfulness versus Supportive Sex Education on Stress in Women with Sexual Interest/Arousal Disorder', *Journal of Behavioral Medicine*, 1–13; Van Minnen, A., and Kampman, M. (2000), 'The Interaction Between Anxiety and Sexual Functioning: A Controlled Study of Sexual Functioning in Women with Anxiety Disorders', *Sexual and Relationship Therapy*, 15(1), 47–57.

NOTES

6 Brotto (2018).
7 Lupien, S., McEwen, B., Gunnar, M. R., and Heim, C. (2009), 'Effects of Stress Throughout the Lifespan on the Brain, Behaviour and Cognition', *Nature Reviews Neuroscience*, 10, 434–45; Brotto (2018), 159; Gurney (2020).
8 Rook, G. A. W., and Stanford, J. L. (1998), 'Give Us This Day Our Daily Germs', *Trends in Immunology*, 19(3), 113–16; Yankouskaya, A., Williamson, R., Stacey, C., Totman, J. J., and Massey, H. (2023), 'Short-Term Head-Out Whole-Body Cold-Water Immersion Facilitates Positive Affect and Increases Interaction Between Large-Scale Brain Networks', *Biology*, 12(2), 211.
9 Burns, D. D. (2007), *When Panic Attacks: The New, Drug-Free Anxiety Therapy That Can Change Your Life*. Harmony.
10 American Psychiatric Association. (2022), 'Depression: What is Depression?', https://psychiatry.org/patients-families/depression/what-is-depression
11 Brotto (2018), 159.
12 Benjet, C., Bromet, E., Karam, E. G., Kessler, R. C., Mclaughlin, K. A., Ruscio, A. M., Shahly, V., Stein, D. J., Petukhova, M., Hill, E., Alonso, J., Atwoli, L., Bunting, B., Bruffaerts, R., Caldas-De-Almeida, J. M., De Girolamo, G., Florescu, S., Gureje, O., Huang, Y., Lepine, J. P., Kawakami, N., Kovess-Masfety, V., Medina-Mora, M. E., Navarro-Mateu, F., Piazza, M., Posada-Villa, J., Scott, K. M., Shalev, A., Slade, T., Ten Have, M., Torres, Y., Viana, M. C., Zarkov, Z., and Koenen, K. C. (2016), 'The Epidemiology of Traumatic Event Exposure Worldwide: Results from the World Mental Health Survey Consortium', *Psychological Medicine*, 46(2), 327–43.

13 Conti, P. (2021), *Trauma: The Invisible Epidemic: How Trauma Works and How We Can Heal from It*, Sounds True, 9.
14 Van Der Kolk, B. A. (2014), *The Body Keeps the Score: Brain, Mind, and Body in the Healing of Trauma*, Viking, 53.
15 Levine, P. A. (1997), *Waking the Tiger: Healing Trauma: The Innate Capacity to Transform Overwhelming Experiences*, North Atlantic Books, 6.
16 Asp, M. (2015), 'Rest: A Health-Related Phenomenon and Concept in Caring Science', *Global Qualitative Nursing Research*, 29(2); Tyler, J. M., and Burns, K. C. (2008), 'After Depletion: The Replenishment of the Self's Regulatory Resources', *Self and Identity*, 7(3), 305–21.
17 Lorde, A. (1988), *A Burst of Light: Essays*, Firebrand Books, 103.
18 Nagoski, E., and Nagoski, A. (2019), *Burnout: The Secret to Unlocking the Stress Cycle*, Ballantine Books, 169.
19 Walker, M. (2018), *Why We Sleep: The New Science of Sleep and Dreams*, Penguin Books.
20 Nagoski and Nagoski (2019), 168.
21 Lembke, A. (2021), *Dopamine Nation: Finding Balance in the Age of Indulgence*, Dutton.
22 Brown, S., and Vaughan, C. (2009), *Play: How It Shapes the Brain, Opens the Imagination, and Invigorates the Soul*, Penguin.
23 Panksepp, J. (2004), *Affective Neuroscience: The Foundations of Human and Animal Emotions*, Oxford University Press.
24 Brown and Vaughan (2009).
25 Perel, E., and Miller, M. A. (2023), 'Letters from Esther #20: Play', https://estherperel.com/blog/letters-from-esther-play.

26 Pellis, S. M., Pellis, V. C., Ham, J. R., and Stark, R. A. (2023), 'Play Fighting and the Development of the Social Brain: The Rat's Tale', *Neuroscience & Biobehavioural Reviews*, 145(105037); Bekoff, M., and Byers, J. A. (eds) (1998), *Animal Play: Evolutionary, Comparative, and Ecological Perspectives*, Cambridge University Press.

27 Panksepp, J. (2004), *Affective Neuroscience: The Foundations of Human and Animal Emotions*, Oxford University Press.

28 Ibid.

29 Brown and Vaughan (2009).

30 Ibid.

31 Fincham, G. W., Strauss, C., Montero-Marin, J., and Cavanagh, K. (2023), 'Effect of Breathwork on Stress and Mental Health: A Meta-analysis of Randomised-Controlled Trials', *Scientific Reports*, 13(1), 432.

32 Khir, M. S., Wan Mohd Yunus, W. W. M. A., Mahmud, N., Wang, R., Panatik, S. A., Mohd Sukor, M. S., and Nordin, N. A. (2024), 'Efficacy of Progressive Muscle Relaxation in Adults for Stress, Anxiety, and Depression: A Systematic Review', *Psychology Research and Behavior Management*, 1(17), 345–65.

33 Brown and Vaughan (2009).

Principle 7 – Prioritize Your Pleasure

1 Hamilton, J. (2021), '11 Kegel Sex Positions for Out-Of-This-World Orgasms: Time to Make Kegel Exercises Your Main Squeeze', *Cosmopolitan*.

2 Thompson, Z. (2016), 'The Incredible Type of Orgasm You Might Be Missing Out On – And How to Have It', *SELF*, https://self.com/story/how-to-have-a-blended-orgasm; Thompson, Z. (2024),

'How to Have Multiple Orgasms When One Just Isn't Enough', *SELF*, https://self.com/story/how-to-have-multiple-orgasms.

3 Gainsburg, M. (2019), 'You Can Totally Have Multiple Orgasms – And It's Easier Than You Think', *Women's Health*, https://womenshealthmag.com/sex-and-love/a28787206/how-to-have-multiple-orgasms/; Hussein, J. (2022), 'Are Extended Orgasms Real? Yes, and Here's How to Make Yours Last Longer: They're Easier to Achieve than You'd Think', *Allure*, https://allure.com/story/extended-orgasms.

4 Herbenick, D., Eastman-Mueller, H., Fu, T. C., Dodge, B., Ponander, K., and Sanders, S. A. (2019), 'Women's Sexual Satisfaction, Communication, and Reasons for (No Longer) Faking Orgasm: Findings from a U.S. Probability Sample', *Archives of Sexual Behavior*, 48(8), 2461–72.

5 Mintz, L. (2018), *Becoming Cliterate: Why Orgasm Equality Matters – And How to Get It*, HarperCollins; Frederick, D. A., John, H. K. S., Garcia, J. R., and Lloyd, E. A. (2018), 'Differences in Orgasm Frequency Among Gay, Lesbian, Bisexual, and Heterosexual Men and Women in a U.S. National Sample', *Archives of Sexual Behavior*, 47(1), 273–88; Wade, L. D., Kremer, E. C., and Brown, J. (2005), 'The Incidental Orgasm: The Presence of Clitoral Knowledge and the Absence of Orgasm for Women', *Women & Health*, 42(1), 117–38; Garcia, J. R., Lloyd, E. A., Wallen, K., and Fisher, H. E. (2014), 'Variation in Orgasm Occurrence by Sexual Orientation in a Sample of U.S. Singles', *Journal of Sexual Medicine*, 11(11), 2645–52; Piemonte, J. L., Conley, T. D., and Gusakova, S. (2019), 'Orgasm, Gender, and Responses to Heterosexual Casual Sex', *Personality and Individual Differences*,

151(109487); Mahar, E. A., Mintz, L. B., and Akers, B. M. (2020), 'Orgasm Equality: Scientific Findings and Societal Implications', *Current Sexual Health Reports*, 12, 24–32; Armstrong, E. A., England, P., and Fogarty, A. C. K. (2012), 'Accounting for Women's Orgasm and Sexual Enjoyment in College Hookups and Relationships', *American Sociological Review*, 77(3), 435–62; Jones, A. C., Robinson, W. D., and Seedall, R. B. (2018), 'The Role of Sexual Communication in Couples' Sexual Outcomes: A Dyadic Path Analysis', *Journal of Marital and Family Therapy*, 44, 606–623; Wetzel, G. M., Cultice, R. A., and Sanchez, D. T. (2022), 'Orgasm Frequency Predicts Desire and Expectation for Orgasm: Assessing the Orgasm Gap Within Mixed-Sex Couples', *Sex Roles*, 86, 456–470.
6 Frederick et al. (2018).
7 Hite, S. (1976), *The Hite Report: A Nationwide Study on Female Sexuality*, Macmillan.
8 Komisaruk, B. R. (2009), *The Orgasm Answer Guide*, The John Hopkins University Press; Mintz (2018).
9 Herbenick, D., Fu, T. C., Arter, J., Sanders, S. A., and Dodge, B. (2018), 'Women's Experiences with Genital Touching, Sexual Pleasure, and Orgasm: Results from a U.S. Probability Sample of Women Ages 18 to 94', *Journal of Sex and Marital Therapy*, 44(2), 201–12.
10 O'Connell, H. E., Hutson, J. M., Anderson, C. R., and Plenter, R. J. (1998), 'Anatomical Relationship Between Urethra and Clitoris', *Journal of Urology*, 159(6), 1892–7; O'Connell, H. E., Sanjeevan, K. V., and Hutson, J. M. (2005), 'Anatomy of the Clitoris', *Journal of Urology*, 174(4 Pt 1), 1189–95.
11 Nagoski (2015).
12 Mintz (2018).

NOTES

13 Ibid.
14 The Cliteracy Project (2015) *The Huffington Post*, https://projects.huffingtonpost.com/projects/cliteracy/embed/history; Longhurst, G. L., Beni, R., Jeong, S. R., Pianta, M., Soper, A. L., Leitch, P., De Witte, G., and Fisher, L. (2023), 'Beyond the Tip of the Iceberg: A Meta-Analysis of the Anatomy of the Clitoris', *Clinical Anatomy* 37(2), 232–52.
15 Institoris, H., Sprenger, J., Koberger, A., and Otto Vollbehr Collection (1494), *Malleus Maleficarum*.
16 Koedt, A. (1970), *The Myth of the Vaginal Orgasm*, New England Free Press.
17 United Nations Children's Fund (2022), 'Female Genital Mutilation (FGM)', https://data.unicef.org/topic/gender/fgm/.
18 Perel, E., and Miller, A. (2023), 'Letters from Esther #37 – Eroticism Is an Art. But It Is Also a Practice', https://estherperel.com/blog/letters-from-esther-37-eroticism-is-an-art-but-its-also-a-practice.
19 Morin, J. (1995), *The Erotic Mind: Unlocking the Inner Sources of Passion and Fulfillment*, HarperCollins.
20 Giddens, A. (1992), *The Transformation of Intimacy: Sexuality, Love and Eroticism in Modern Societies*, Polity Press.
21 Lorde, A. (1978), 'Uses of the Erotic: The Erotic as Power', Paper Delivered at The Fourth Berkshire Conference on The History of Women, Mount Holyoke College, August 25, 1978, in *Sister Outsider: Essays and Speeches by Audre Lorde*, Crossing Press.
22 Morin (1995), 2.
23 Brotto (2018); Paterson, L. Q. P., Handy, A. B., and Brotto, L. A. (2017), 'A Pilot Study of Eight-Session Mindfulness-Based Cognitive Therapy Adapted for

Women's Sexual Interest/Arousal Disorder', *Journal of Sex Research*, 54(7), 850–61.

24 Kleinplatz, P. J., and Ménard, A. D. (2020), *Magnificent Sex: Lessons from Extraordinary Lovers*, Routledge/Taylor & Francis Group; Barker, M. J., and Hancock, J. (2017), *Enjoy Sex: How, When and If You Want To*, Icon Books.

25 Nhât Hanh, T. (1999), *The Miracle of Mindfulness: An Introduction to the Practice of Meditation*, Beacon Press.

26 Kabat-Zinn, J. (1994), *Wherever You Go, There You Are: Mindfulness Meditation in Everyday Life*, Piatkus.

27 Brotto (2018).

28 Morone, N. E., Greco, C. M., Moore, C. G., Rollman, B. L., Lane, B., Morrow, L. A., Glynn, N. W., and Weiner, D. K. (2016), 'A Mind-Body Program for Older Adults with Chronic Low Back Pain: A Randomized Clinical Trial', *JAMA Internal Medicine*, 176(3), 329–37; Cherkin, D. C., Sherman, K. J., Balderson, B. H., Cook, A. J., Anderson, M. L., Hawkes, R. J., Hansen, K. E., and Turner, J. A. (2016), 'Effect of Mindfulness-Based Stress Reduction Vs Cognitive Behavioral Therapy or Usual Care on Back Pain and Functional Limitations in Adults with Chronic Low Back Pain: A Randomized Clinical Trial', *JAMA*, 315(12), 1240–49; Hofmann, S. G., Sawyer, A. T., Witt, A. A., and Oh, D. (2010), 'The Effect of Mindfulness-Based Therapy on Anxiety and Depression: A Meta-Analytic Review', *Journal of Consulting and Clinical Psychology*, 78(2), 169–83; Segal, Z. V., Williams, J. M. G., and Teasdale, J. D. (2002), *Mindfulness-Based Cognitive Therapy for Depression: A New Approach to Preventing Relapse*, Guilford Press; Jaderek, I., and Lew-Starowicz, M. (2019), 'A Systematic Review on Mindfulness Meditation-Based Interventions for

Sexual Dysfunctions', *Journal of Sexual Medicine*, 16(10), 1581–96.
29 Brotto (2018).
30 Paterson, L. Q. P., Handy, A. B., and Brotto, L. A. (2017), 'A Pilot Study of Eight-Session Mindfulness-Based Cognitive Therapy Adapted for Women's Sexual Interest/Arousal Disorder', *Journal of Sex Research*, 54(7), 850–61.
31 Bryant, F. B., and Joseph Veroff, J. (2017), *Savouring: A New Model of Positive Experience*, Taylor & Francis.
32 Herlin, B., Leu-Semescu, S., Chaumereuil, C., and Arnulf, I. (2015), 'Evidence That Non-Dreamers Do Dream: A REM Sleep Behaviour Disorder Model', *Journal of Sleep Research*, 24(6), 602–9.
33 Perel (2007).
34 Lehmiller, J. J. (2020), *Tell Me What You Want: The Science of Sexual Desire and How It Can Help You Improve Your Sex Life*, Hachette.
35 Kahr, B. (2008), *Who's Been Sleeping In Your Head?: The Secret World of Sexual Fantasies*, Basic Books.
36 Morin (1995).
37 Perel, E., and Miller, M. A. (2023), 'Why Do Sexual Taboos Make Up Our Sexual Fantasies?', https://estherperel.com/blog/sexual-taboos-sexual-fantasy.
38 Bader, M. J. (2003), *Arousal: The Secret Logic of Fantasies*, Macmillan.
39 Brotto (2018).

Principle 8 – Improve Your Communication

1 Gottman, J. M. (1994), *What Predicts Divorce? The Relationship Between Marital Processes and Marital Outcomes*, Lawrence Erlbaum Associates.

NOTES

2 Hunkins, A. (2022), 'The #1 Obstacle to Effective Communication', *Forbes*; Corbett, H. (2023), '3 Ways to Manage Conflict in the Workplace', *Forbes*.
3 Stone, D., Patton, B., and Heen, S. (2010), *Difficult Conversations: How to Discuss What Matters Most*, Penguin.
4 Stone, D., and Heen, S. (2015), *Thanks for the Feedback: The Science and Art of Receiving Feedback Well*, Penguin, 18.
5 Davidson, R., and Begley, S. (2012), *The Emotional Life of Your Brain: How Its Unique Patterns Affect the Way You Think, Feel and Live – And How You Can Change Them*, Avery.
6 Weitzel, S. (2007), *Feedback That Works: How to Build and Deliver Your Message*, Center for Creative Leadership, Wiley.

Conclusion

1 Carroll, L. (1993) *Alice's Adventures in Wonderland*, Dover Publications.

Index

adrenaline 136, 200, 208
agency, asserting 17–19,
    29–35, 40–49, 315
    see also boundaries
alcohol 54, 209, 210
*Alice's Adventures in
    Wonderland* 15, 213
all-or-nothing thinking
    106, 117
amber flags 89
anhedonia 203
anorgasmia xii, 241
antidepressants 198
anxiety 10, 22–3, 159, 192,
    197, 203
    and attachment
    147
apathy 197
apologising 295–6
Apple xiii
arguments *see* conflict
arousal 160, 168, 174
    hyper-arousal 200–201
    non-concordance 176,
        190, 316

physical and mental
    175–6
attachment styles 125–6,
    129, 155–6
    and building intimacy
    147–50
    insecure 129–33, 137,
    147–9
    quiz 143–7
    secure 130, 134, 137,
    139–41, 149–50
Attachment Theory in Practice
    141
autoimmune diseases 204

Basson, Rosemary 167, 193
Bates, Laura 63
BDSM 250
beliefs 104–5
    limiting 3, 121
    reframing 114–16
beta blockers 198
biology 9–10
    and desire 164–5
blaming 31, 108, 292

INDEX

The Body Keeps the Score 204
body language 278, 281
body mapping 181–7, 316
boundaries 48, 197
   asserting 23, 25–6
   flexible 28–9, 41–2
   healthy 33–5
   physical space 33, 43
   porous 26–7, 40–42
   rigid 27–8, 41–2, 132
   setting 19, 40–45
   and touching 186
brain, and sexual response 135–6, 168–9, 173–5, 251
break-ups 36–7, 162
breathwork 221–3, 246–7, 316
Brotto, Lori 176, 193
Brown, Brené xiv, 7
Brown, Stuart 212, 214
bullying 22
Bumble 22, 198, 217
burnout 27, 207, 235

cancer 206
catastrophizing 107, 117
catcalls 22
censorship xiii
change, fallacy of 108
childhood 94–5, 129, 290
children 33, 166, 194, 284, 286, 306

Chivers, Meredith 174, 193
chlamydia 38
chronic fatigue syndrome 204
cisgender experience 14–15
class, social 15, 59
clitoris 185, 239–41, 264–6
co-dependence 27
coercion 61
cognitive distortions 106–9, 122
   challenging 116–18
Come As You Are 169, 240
commitment 147
communication 69, 83, 317
   and boundaries 43–5
   confident 270–312
   learning 277–312
   and repairing relationships 295–8
compliance, sexual 32, 37
condoms 38–9
confidence 1–2, 19, 99, 121
   building 91–2, 114–22, 315
   in communicating 270–312
conflict 147, 272
   healthy 295–302
consent 18–19, 49, 52
   and agency 30–31
   and arousal 176–7
   and pressure or threats 31

INDEX

contempt 67–9, 89
Conti, Paul 204
contraception 18, 30, 38–9
conversations about sex
   270–312
  difficult 279–83
coping strategies 82
core beliefs 104–5
  reframing 114–16
creativity 210
criticism 66, 69, 81
cuddling 126, 211
culture
  and core beliefs 105
  influence on sex 9–10,
   233

dating 139–40
daydreams 249
decision-making 39, 46–7,
  52, 81–2
defensiveness 65, 67, 69,
  81, 89
dependency 148
depression 192, 193, 197,
  203
desire
  body mapping 181–7,
   316
  and the brain 168–73
  creating an inventory
   180–81
  as depicted in films 158

  embracing 158–61,
   177–91, 316
  expressing 302–4
  gender differences
   167–8
  low 6, 159–61, 166, 178,
   193, 203, 241
  mismatched 178–9
  physiological responses
   173–5
  products for boosting
   170–71
  responsive 190
  stimuli for 167–8
Diazepam 198
digital harassment 62
disability 18, 59
disassociation 198
divorce 124
dopamine 135, 172, 174,
  239, 254
Dopamine Nation 207
drains vs gains 86–7
dreams 249
drugs 209
dryness 24

Eisenhower Matrix 39,
  46–7
embarrassment 4, 44, 260
empathy 71, 119
encouragement 83
endorphins 174

INDEX

erection problems 271, 274
erotica 35, 216, 260–61
eroticism 233–4, 317
   in everyday life 1, 256–7
   exploring 243–6
   and meditation 259–60
Escape the City 75, 111
exercise 194, 210
extroverts 135

fairness, fallacy of 108
fantasies 24, 179, 216, 249–52, 257–9, 267–8, 317
fear of sexuality 57, 76
feedback 271, 283–8, 304–7
   effective 291–5
feminism 15
Ferly app xi–xiii, 4, 113, 241, 249, 299–300
fibromyalgia 204
films, depicting desire 158
financial abuse 62
flirting 94
food 208, 210
foreplay 29, 39, 183
   skipping 27–8
Freud, Sigmund 165, 240
future, manifesting 118–19

gaming 209
gaslighting 63–5

gender differences 52, 93–5, 101, 270
gender identity 14, 18
generalization 106
genital mutilation 241
genitals xii, 6, 176, 240, 261, 264
   touching 185–6
   see also clitoris
Giddens, Anthony 244
Glover Tawwab, Nedra 38
goals 4, 17, 71, 82–3, 120
Goss, Charles Mayo 240
Gottman, John 65–6, 69, 271
Gottman, Julie 271
gratitude 83, 152–4, 186
green flags 70–72, 89
Grey's Anatomy 240–41
Gurney, Karen 165

harassment 62
health and wellbeing 193
   caring for 9, 199–200, 206, 209–10, 316
   tools for 221–4
heart-to-hearts 83
heaven's reward 108
Hite Report 233
honesty 13
hugging 33, 274
humiliation 67

INDEX

identity, talking about 282–3, 285, 288
illness 166
imposter syndrome 139
intimacy
   and attachment styles 129–34
   building 147–56
   cultivating 123–5, 136–43, 207, 316
   inventory of needs 150–52
introverts 135

Johnson, Sue 141
joy, auditing 85, 87
judgement, fear of 92

Kabat-Zinn, Jon 247
Kennedy, Becky 38
kintsugi 199
kissing 28, 126–7, 182, 274

labelling 108
Lehmiller, Justin 250
Lembke, Anna 207
Levine, Peter 204
LGBTQIA+ community 14, 192, 233
libido 165, 170–71, 241
light, natural 210
limiting beliefs 3, 121
Lloyd, Elisabeth 239

loneliness 135–6
Lorde, Audre 206, 244
Los Angeles 235–6
Lust, Erika 179

manifesting 118–20
marriage 115, 123
massage 119, 168, 179, 184, 215, 228, 263
masturbation 3, 111, 179, 207, 210
   and self-pleasure 262–5
   shame about 111
Mating in Captivity 172, 249–50
meditation 184, 248, 254–6
   erotic 259–60
men, experience of desire 167
Men Who Hate Women 63
menopause 166
mental filtering 106
mental health 9–10, 316
   breakdowns 198, 217–20
   impact on sex 193–4, 202–5
   medication 198
   see also anxiety; depression; panic attacks; trauma
me-time 82
Miller, Alice 241

Miller, Mary Alice 142
mindfulness 1, 246–8, 250, 256, 262, 317
Mintz, Laurie 233
misogyny 63
mockery 67
monogamy 215
Morin, Jack 246

Nagoski, Emily 167, 169, 172, 207, 239–40
nervous system 230
   balanced 200–203
non-binary experience 14
norepinephrine 173

O'Connell, Helen 239
Omeprazole 198
oral sex 45, 126
orgasms 3, 232–3, 238–9, 241–3, 317
   faking 27, 95, 117, 233
   and gender differences 6, 233
overplanning 208
oxytocin 174, 239

pain, during sex xii, 24, 27, 159, 202
panic attacks 195–6
partners, checking in with 29, 83–5
peeping Toms 22

penetration, painful xii, 24
penis 239–40
people-pleasing 36, 276
Perel, Esther 142, 172, 241, 249
performance anxiety 241
photographs, explicit 23
physical space 33
play 211–16, 266
   and fantasies 251
   personalities 213–14, 224–9
   and sex 212–13, 215–16
pleasure 174
   focusing on 233–4, 241–6
   lack of 197
   losing 235–7
   and masturbation 262–5
   and orgasms 232–3
   prioritising 238–9, 253–67, 317
   as a right 9
   and self-care 212–13
   self-pleasuring 210, 220, 262, 265, 317
pop culture 158–9, 167
porn 170, 207, 254
   ethical 260
   overuse 209
power 67
   green flags 70–72

imbalances 51–8, 77,
    87–8, 315
'power over' 58–9,
    63–5, 88
'power to' 60, 68, 77, 88
'power with' 60–61, 70,
    88
quiz 77–81
red flags 61–2, 65, 88
shared 70
privilege 59
projecting 64

race 15, 18, 59, 93
rape 20–22, 31, 89
    by partners 31
red flags 61–2, 65, 88
reflection 304–7
relationships
    and communication
        270–312
    healthy 71, 82–4
    professional/working
        299–300
    repairing 296–7
relaxation 223–4
resilience 71
resources 11
rest 206–11, 218
    distractions from
        207–9
retreats 235–6, 254
retrospectives 83–5

risk-taking 100, 208
role play 215–16
romance 127–8

same-sex relationships
    52, 233
sarcasm 67
satisfaction 124, 128, 135,
    166, 207, 243, 271–2,
    311
screen time 208, 210
self-confidence *see*
    confidence
self-discovery 1, 113, 150,
    252, 313–14, 320–21
self-efficacy 99, 102–3,
    121, 315
self-esteem 99–101, 121,
    315
self-touch 185–6, 210
The Seven Principles for
    Making Marriage Work
    65–6
sex
    aversion to 3
    detachment from 20
    as a drive 164–6
    expressing needs
        302–4
    fear of sexuality 57, 76
    motivation for 164–7,
        180, 190, 192
    parties 215

sex – *cont'd.*
  as play 212–13, 215–16
  toys 111, 170, 215,
    260–61
  unwanted and lack of
    32, 37, 162, 274
sexting 23
sexual assault ix, xi, 53–4,
  71, 163, 204
  impact on desire 163
sexual excitation system
  (SES) 169
sexual inhibition system
  (SIS) 169
sexual orientation 18, 52
shame xiii–xiv, 6–7, 13,
  111, 127, 260
shopping 208
'should' statements 107
shyness 4
Silver, Nan 65
Situation, Behaviour,
  Impact and Action
  (SBIA) 291–5, 312,
  317
sleep 198, 200–201, 206–7,
  209, 218, 249
social activity 210, 214
social bonds 136, 214
solo time 82
somatic bodywork 7
'spark' in relationships
  159

spontaneity 159, 163,
  167–8, 190, 193
stalking 62, 88
stonewalling 68–9, 89, 290
storytelling 216
stress 10, 136, 166, 192
  good 202
sulking 31, 68, 128
supplements 170–71
swinging 215

taboos 6, 10, 251
talking, about sex 270–312
tantra 7
teamwork 83
TEDx 113
therapy 38, 65, 198, 218
Thích Nhất Hạnh 247
tiredness and fatigue 204
touch 34, 111, 141, 182,
  185–9, 210, 220,
  263–6, 274, 289, 297,
  303
trans experience 14
trauma 3, 89, 148, 197,
  204–5
triggers 285–91, 301

vagina xii, 6, 176, 185, 240,
  264
vaginismus xii, 176
validation, seeking 110,
  117, 131

values 17, 119, 183
van der Kolk, Bessel 204
Vesalius, Andreas 240
vibrators 35, 111, 207, 210
violence, sexual ix, 21–2, 204, 215, 260
   in the workplace 53–4, 73–6
   see also rape
vulnerability xiv, 28, 150, 205, 272
vulvodynia xii

Weitzel, Sloan 291
wellbeing 193
   caring for 9, 199–200, 206, 209–10, 316
   tools for 221–4
work 34, 92, 208
workplace violence 53–4, 73–6
World Health Organization (WHO) 8–9

Zinc VC ix–x